Peer Review, Peer Education, and Modeling in the Practice of Clinical Ethics Consultation: The Zadeh Project

Stuart G. Finder • Mark J. Bliton
Editors

Peer Review, Peer Education, and Modeling in the Practice of Clinical Ethics Consultation: The Zadeh Project

Springer Open

Editors
Stuart G. Finder
Center for Healthcare Ethics
Cedars-Sinai Medical Center
Los Angeles, CA, USA

Mark J. Bliton
Medical Bioethics
Kaiser Permanente Los Angeles
Medical Center
Los Angeles, CA, USA

ISBN 978-3-030-08140-9 ISBN 978-3-319-90955-4 (eBook)
https://doi.org/10.1007/978-3-319-90955-4

Printed on acid-free paper

This Springer imprint is published by the registered company Springer Nature Switzerland AG
The registered company address is: Gewerbestrasse 11, 6330 Cham, Switzerland

To Jim Sheridan, who taught and guided each of us into the world of philosophy; to Dick Zaner, our mentor, friend, and colleague-in-arms whose orientation and work continues to direct us into the wonder and awe of the clinical encounter; and to our parents – Moses and Laryn, Katheryn and Jerry – and wives – Cindy and Amy – and children – Jackson, Sam, Sarah, Nathan, and Chloe – whose love and embrace encourages us daily to step forward into the unfolding mysteries . . . and discover.

Acknowledgments

It is with deep and abiding gratitude that we thank all of our colleagues who have participated in the Zadeh Project. Having been involved in the field of clinical ethics for quite some time (well over a quarter century now), we are quite aware that sustained engagement of the kind we have sought throughout this Project is not the norm. Indeed, the amount of time that has passed since we began the effort to unfold this project – starting as it did when we initially sent the Zadeh Scenario to our first set of collaborators to probe nearly a decade ago and lasting until the event of this current publication – reflects perseverance and a willingness to trust; such is not to be taken for granted.

Equally deserving of explicit recognition are the many patients and families with whom we have been privileged to participate in the course of both our shared and separate clinical work. These interactions have brought us into some of the most intimate and gravest moments that individuals experience – such as those involving discussions about the end of a specific person's life. Especially to those who opened their lives in hopes of assisting the rest of us to better face such moments in our own lives, we are truly indebted and grateful.

In addition to those we have acknowledged above, our gratitude to Mrs. Hamadani, her son Samir Zadeh, her daughters Nadira and Farzana, Dr. Brouhkim, and the other individuals presented in "The Zadeh Scenario" cannot be overstated. While names and identifying information have been altered so as to protect privacy, their story is accurate in its core moral, ethical, and medical details as are those additional and more far reaching social and human dimensions taken up by this book.

Contents

INTRODUCTION

The Zadeh Project – A Frame for Understanding the Generative Ideas, Formation, and Design

Mark J. Bliton and Stuart G. Finder

> *"Taking things for granted" is a phrase which, taken literally, would be morally legitimate if we realized that this was really a "grant," an unearned gift.*
>
> Herbert Speigelberg (1975)

Ideas Behind the Initiation of the Zadeh Project

This book represents a unique contribution to the field of clinical ethics consultation. What might seem at first glance to be an anthology, that is, a collection of independent essays, is actually more akin to a conversation, a shared engagement, a mutual undertaking. At the center of this conversation is a steadfastness, abiding and serious in its orientation – exemplified in these voices and contributions collected from colleagues – to explore, identify, and examine the actual conduct of individuals who engage in ethics consultation practice. Although there is some helpful resemblance to an anthology, for example in the variety of ways these essays describe and depict a complex array of different standpoints regarding the practical and conceptual commitments in this growing field, more important to the Zadeh Project is the deliberate focus on explicating and probing the ways these commitments influence how a particular individual acting as an "ethics consultant" might understand and interpret the roles and prevalent expectations represented by those differing standpoints. In that light, and perhaps more urgently, this book is motivated by a mutual recognition that part and parcel with the responsibility of doing

M. J. Bliton (✉)
Medical Bioethics, Kaiser Permanente Los Angeles Medical Center, Los Angeles, CA, USA
e-mail: Mark.J.Bliton@kp.org

S. G. Finder
Center for Healthcare Ethics, Cedars-Sinai Medical Center, Los Angeles, CA, USA
e-mail: Stuart.Finder@cshs.org

S. G. Finder, M. J. Bliton (eds.), *Peer Review, Peer Education, and Modeling in the Practice of Clinical Ethics Consultation: The Zadeh Project*,
https://doi.org/10.1007/978-3-319-90955-4_1

clinical ethics is an ongoing and clear need to describe and consider what clinical ethics consultants actually encounter when actively working with physicians, nurses, social workers, and other healthcare providers as well as with patients, families, and others who care about patients. As a contribution to that necessity of being accountable, this Project and the resulting book represent much more than merely collecting together the thoughts and perspectives of a group of colleagues from within a common field: this book is an attempt to display, to model through written text, a set of practices and what is at stake in these practices.

Like any collective effort of this sort, the Zadeh Project has a history and context that situates the story of its development. It began, first and foremost, with an actual clinical ethics consultation, after which, as part of the effort to reflect on what had occurred during that consultation episode, words were committed to the page and the end result was a manuscript: the Zadeh Scenario developed and written by Stuart Finder (2018). The Project also grew out of our previous investigations, writing, and publications regarding a central idea: writing about clinical ethics consultations can be – and more importantly needs to be – understood as a form of inquiry, even discovery, about the facts, perspectives, commitments, and interpretations regarding what is most worthwhile to those people most intimately involved in what are typically called "ethics cases" (Bliton and Finder 2002; Bliton 2005; Finder and Bliton 2008, 2011). Throughout this Project, the Zadeh Scenario has thus served as the touchstone, the independent variable, if you will, that remains constant. The text for this Scenario was not edited nor revised over the course of this Project. It has remained intact, word for word (several typos, understandably, were corrected prior to publication here) as initially written and then shared, first with Bliton, as part of Finder's effort to gain some understanding about the experience it captures. In this way, the Zadeh Scenario has served as the locus for primary examination and critical interpretation from the start.

Using the Zadeh Scenario in this way demonstrates another prominent theme for this book, namely, that the clinical and moral work of clinical ethics consultation is primarily communicative, involving many varied forms of telling and listening which thereby elicit additional repetitions, including written forms, to establish clearly, to the extent possible, what is morally relevant (Zaner 1993, 1998, 2004a, b). This kind of repetition and focused examination was modeled throughout the different stages of the Zadeh Project, including the design and format for the book. The Project began in earnest when we first solicited critical views from colleagues beyond our own immediate group, colleagues who represent a considerable range among contemporary standpoints regarding clinical ethics.

Specifically, the discussions that formed the Zadeh Project were initially carried out in a series of presentations conducted at several national and international Bioethics and clinical ethics consultation conferences. The first was a panel discussion at the *6th International Conference on Clinical Ethics Consultation,* in Portland, Oregon, during May 2010. Encouraged by the response we received from both our collaborators for that panel and the audience who attended the presentation, in 2012 at the *14th Annual Meeting of the American Society for Bioethics and Humanities,* then again with a different set of colleagues in 2013 at the *9th International Conference on Clinical Ethics Consultation* at Klinikum Ludwig-Maximillians-University in Munich, Germany, we conducted extended workshops in order to examine more fully the complex set of themes which emerged in the initial panel, namely, themes regarding moral experiences encountered in "doing" ethics consultation as well as the sort of assessments encountered in peer review. In all three professional presentations, we explicitly told our colleagues who presented with us and those in the audience that the Zadeh Scenario manuscript was being used to evoke, to allude to, to bring into the discourse with our audiences a recognition of the varieties and different modes of communication that often emerge in clinical discussions about what really matters to the people involved.

More importantly, especially for the two workshops, we engaged in these explorations with an explicit acknowledgement of our own commitment to examine those frequent occasions in which the words, interactions, and different ways of "listening and talking" in clinical encounters are key indications about what matters in the experiences of those people most intimately and personally involved. Indeed, then as now, we acknowledged that from the very moment ethics consultants begin interacting with a patient, a family, or other healthcare professionals, those same ethics consultants may come into direct contact with experiences that are frequently overwhelming to these other persons' lives. What is required from ethics consultants, especially at the very beginning of such interactions, therefore, is a careful and practical kind of listening and talking by which to identify and measure how to help those others think about their own beliefs and values, and to help these people understand the issues posed by their own circumstances, as well as to help them anticipate, and then consider, the ways to best face their circumstances in the present and going forward into the future. As Richard Zaner puts it, to "enter a clinical situation is invariably to encounter a multitude of voices – at times muted, at others pleading, at times a veritable cacophony" (Zaner 1998: 69). "Working within such a resounding legion of voices," Zaner says elsewhere, "is surely one of the most striking factors about being involved as an ethicist in clinical encounters" (Zaner 2015: 114). "Thus," he continues, "the image of 'voices' – challenging, compelling, urgently seeking to be heard – and the exigencies of time – time to think about matters, time to speak and be heard, time to listen, time to settle disputed things" are themes that run through every clinical encounter (Zaner 2015: 114).

The panel and subsequent workshops were thus designed around this focus on careful and practical listening and talking in order to raise, explicitly, these themes of voices and time in discussions about clinical ethics. Likewise, these were designed to examine deliberately whether, and to what extent, these integral activities of talking and listening are recognized as essential for the practices of clinical consultation about ethics. The idea, in keeping with Zaner's "multitude of voices," was that such talking and listening consists in recognizing the interests and attention, the threats, agreements, expectations, memories, indications, faith, suspicions, trust, even promises and deceptions, of those individuals immediately involved in a particular clinical situation.

We therefore conducted all three of these conference-based sessions with different groups of ethics consultants and Bioethics colleagues – this too was a deliberate and intentional way to explore how discussions that are conversational and in person, as exemplified by participation in those conference settings, provide immediate examples and reflect (or not) typical assumptions about roles, participation, subject-matter content, context of interaction, and so on. Of course, such assumptions inform and yet also limit both the type and extent of clarifications that may occur in professional discourse. For example, topics in clinical ethics, or Bioethics more generally – for instance, discussions about a patient's dying or decisions to limit the provision of medical interventions – are assumed to be similar across settings or contexts. What we sought to explore are the ways that contexts, presuppositions, and roles may be relevantly *different* in these different circumstances; for example, when participating on a Medical Center Task Force or in institutional committee meetings, the vocabularies, the conversational tone, and length of time spent to explain the moral contents and practical implications may be quite different from expressions used for those same elements during clinical meetings with patients, providers, family members, and so on. Therefore, recognizing and responding to differences among these kinds of activities becomes crucial to clinical ethics practice in health care environments. Moreover, the meanings of ethics topics, their presuppositions, and the vocabularies used must be understood as directly correlated to the specific kind of circumstances *and* the specific kind of attention directed *to* those circumstances – which serves to distinguish what is relevant and what is not (Schutz 1967a: 73).[1]

The same need to distinguish relevant differences among related activities would thus seem to arise when called to understand and respond to writing in or about clinical ethics, e.g., an ethics consultant's personal notes, chart notes, case presentations, and so on.[2] These activities organize different kinds of documentation. They divide it up, create some order for it, even arrange it among various levels, including the distribution of what is written in different contexts across time. This need to

[1]Following Schutz, Richard Zaner (Zaner 1988, 1998, 2004b, 2006), and others like Arthur Kleinman (Kleinman 1988, 2006) and Arthur Frank (Frank 1997, 2001) show the ways clinical medicine and clinical ethics embody entire sets of deeply sedimented assumptions about multiple roles and interactions, which themselves presuppose additional theories about interpersonal relations and communication. Given that any adequate examination of the methodologies needed to understand these social, clinical, and interpersonal relationships, and communications would require a daunting combination of wide-ranging conceptual and empirical studies, there is much work that remains to be done, although there have been significant contributions made in a number of specific enclaves which inform the activities of clinical ethics consultation (See, Starr 1982; Zussman 1992; Anspach 1995; Fox and Swazey 2008; Bosk 2009; Evans 2012; Kaufman 2015).

[2]For example, the topic of writing and placing of a chart note in the medical record represents consistent focus for discourse, argument, and claims made about the relevance of clinical ethics consultation to the identification, clarification and resolution of moral issues in health care. These arguments and claims have continued throughout the development of the field (see Freedman 1993). Nancy Dubler and the Working Group for the Clinical Ethics Credentialing Project have made charting the centerpiece of their argument for credentialing clinical ethics consultants, (see Dubler et al. 2009; Bruce et al. 2014).

distinguish holds even more pointedly for writing intended as a critical or interpretive commentary about a particular situation, topic, or theme for professional presentation and publication.

Therefore, another question we put to our collaborators as part of those conference presentations – and which we similarly asked of the contributors for this *written* version of the Zadeh Project – was to consider just how – that is, in what ways – would those interactive elements of ethics consultation, documentation, and various forms of writing figure into and be accounted for in peer review?[3] After all, among the most serious questions that any ethicist must engage, surely one primary task is that of finding the best way, and to employ the most faithful way, to express the complex range and scope of moral considerations that are generated as well as evoked throughout ethics consultation work (Chambers 2000; Molewijk et al. 2016).

Building upon what we experienced and learned from doing the panel in Portland back in 2010 and then in the subsequent workshops in 2012 and 2013, this book is designed to solicit and explore just these kinds of practical issues that emerge among the multiple explanations about the moral experiences and content encountered when "doing" ethics consultation – as well as to solicit and explore what *else* might be learned about such "doing."[4] Accordingly, the variety of assumptions and assessments presented by the essays published here may be taken as representing additional ways to understand Zaner's recognition of the challenging and compelling voices that need to be heard. Accordingly, there is no single, determinate story or authoritative voice in this Zadeh Project. Instead, it presents a mosaic composed of diverse standpoints, multiple variations expressing similar and related themes, and generates a manifold of questions and different voices, as well as valuable criticisms. These, of course, all need more explicit and careful investigation as the field of clinical ethics consultation grapples with the demands of personal and professional obligations inherent to clinical work and the extensive scope of professional responsibilities that confront future development. The Zadeh Project, therefore, is not designed to provide definitive answers but to evoke and provide some shape for pertinent questions and inquiry.

For our own part, we maintain that these recognitions and responsibilities are generated in the necessary and crucial influence of the "clinical turn" in ethics, which has been exemplified in the work and publications by Zaner and others (Zaner 1988, 2006; Andre 2002; Churchill et al. 2013). This "clinical turn" demonstrates the need to pay explicit attention to what is commonplace, the taken-for-granted in everyday life, and reveals how it is *there* that moral experience and ethical significance are rooted (Zaner 1984; Hoffmaster 1992). Having taken that 'turn,' not only are we quite cognizant of the variety of ways the roles for clinical ethics are

[3] Proposals have been published recently by a number of scholars, (see discussions in Fins et al. 2016 and Pearlman et al. 2016).

[4] In this sense, the Zadeh Project may be placed alongside such previous efforts as Andre 2002; Zaner 2004a; Ford and Dudzinski 2008.

conceptualized,[5] but we are committed to maintaining such diversity of expression. Such is the grounding frame for the Zadeh Project and hence this book.

A Brief Explanation of the Method Used in the Design for the Zadeh Project

In light of the groundwork and frame discussed above, this book is organized around a practical feature of professional life that sociologist Harold Garfinkel termed a "documentary method of interpretation" (Garfinkel 1967: 76–103). With roots in the work of Alfred Schutz and Aron Gurwitsch in phenomenology and social psychology, the "documentary method of interpretation" uses the idea that in ordinary everyday life what we experience is typically understood as presenting or reflecting underlying (and presupposed) patterns of belief, expectations for interactions, and their meanings.[6] To better understand what others hold to be worthwhile requires probing with them what is at stake, what is most cherished within those beliefs, identifiable values, stories, and situations that are presented as meaningful. This rationale provides the key to following the development of explanations and critiques throughout the sections and chapters that compose this book, and likewise provides a way to integrate and make sense of the observations and themes gathered from one chapter or another by reference to that larger context of the Zadeh Project.

As mentioned above, the unaltered Zadeh Scenario has remained the touchstone throughout this Project. Therefore, a specific set of observations by one author using, for example, a conversation between Finder and the patient's daughters, or the dialogue between Finder and Dr. Broukhim can be seen as a document – or in other words, an instance of – a manifestation, possibly a symptom or an indication, of a particular kind of issue. And, the variations among the ways that these instances are discussed in the different contributions can be compared in order to identify those additional assumptions used by these authors to create and support an assessment of clinical ethics consultation.

---

[5] The breadth of different concepts may be found in such works as Jecker et al. 2012; Gaines and Juengst 2008; Aulisio et al. 2003; Engelhardt 1996; Jonsen and Toulmin 1988.

[6] For Garfinkel, the initial conception and development for this method was for conducting the work of social scientific studies, in which Garfinkel elaborated on Schutz's interest and insight regarding the ways that schemes of relevance are used in what Garfinkel called "common sense knowledge of social structures" (Garfinkel 1967: 76). Likewise, Schutz's explication of sociality has been decisive for Zaner's investigations into many enclaves of meaning in clinical medicine and clinical ethics, for example the relationships among physicians and patients, the illness experience of patients – as interpreted by patients, then physicians and others, the core moral elements of responsibility, and the imperative to not take advantage of patients (see especially Zaner 2004b). More specifically, a theme prominent for Zaner, and for the Zadeh Project, pertains to those communicative dimensions where Zaner so brilliantly extends Schutz's ideas about "face-to-face" and the attitudes of "taken-for-grantedness" into his own investigations of moral and clinical life.

This method thus serves as a key because it enables the readers to trace out various responses to those issues, as well as the interpretive themes that emerge among the essays. Likewise, this method demonstrates the similarities and critical differences among the ways this Zadeh Scenario is read by the contributors, specifically in the way that several direct their focus on procedures and rules, thereby documenting implications for the meanings assigned to 'ethics', as well as the different ways the range of questions and issues are presented.

To help frame that crucial topic which focuses on rules and procedures for ethics consultation, consider one widely used conception of clinical ethics employed when ethical troubles or "problems" arise. Where these troubles call for a response, the role of clinical ethics consultation is to operationalize the way healthcare institutions respond to these "problems" (Curtis et al. 2012; Nelson 2010; Foglia 2012). In addition, this view illustrates a tendency in writing about clinical ethics. Problems, issues, concerns, and topics are called "ethical" in ways that do not seem to have faced or, at a minimum, are remote from the bristling thicket of emotions and face-to-face interactions that frequently provide clues to identifying those values that people hold most worthwhile in clinical situations (Komesaroff 2001; Molewijk et al. 2011). The characteristic assumption at the organizational level is that the function, the job, of ethics consultation is to make those sorts of problems recognizable as "typical," and then to use standardized expectations, policies, norms, and so on to explain how and why to respond (Frank 2004; Bruce et al. 2015).

With that reliance on standardized expectations, policies, and procedures for conducting clinical ethics consultations, the focus shifts from talking about the moral reasons and actions that prompted those expectations, policies, procedures and so on, in the first place to the effective fulfillment or completion of the designated procedures, so that "ethics" becomes a set of procedures performed in an accountable way.[7]

The "documentary method" used throughout this book therefore provides a practical means by which to identify and interrogate – with a degree of rigor appropriate to the level of investigation – what is morally at stake in, and possibly neglected by, that complex network of discrete and multiple forms of communication and interactions in clinical situations (Natanson 1970; Zaner 1981; Rogers 1983). This method

[7] The significance of this substantive and practical issue becomes powerfully evident when we realize, as discussed by Alasdair MacIntyre in his generative book, *After Virtue* (MacIntyre 1984), that in a pluralistic society like ours there are not only any number of different ethical viewpoints, but that these are deeply at odds with each other. Although each of them may be perfectly self-consistent, each starts from quite different basic premises that rival others. Thus, substantive moral problems continue to arise when "ethics" is used as the means to "fill in the appropriate 'moral' or 'values' stance" category in a procedure authorized by an organization. The typical, and expected, result is to "manage" the problem by the ethics consultant determining which of the competing values or viewpoints is to be authorized to rule in the clinical decision or negotiation. In the case of conflict between two different standpoints, momentous problems arise, because such conflict resists being resolved equitably, due to that lack of a coherent rule of judgment applicable to both standpoints. Of course, rules can be, and indeed are, stipulated that a consultant simply 'follows the procedure' to create a result. The effect, however, merely documents another standpoint in conflict with the ones that this procedure is intended to resolve, and so on.

can thus be used to investigate additional organizational attitudes and beliefs that underwrite those expectations, norms, and interactions.

In that context, another rationale for utilizing this method as a key component of the Zadeh Project involves an analogy used by Zaner (whose work is deeply rooted in the same phenomenological tradition as that of Schutz, Gurwitsch, and Garfinkel). Zaner's idea is that a clinical ethics consultant works like a sort of clinical detective, and as an interpreter of those "texts" and "documents" created amidst that confluence of individuals, relationships, interactions, and environments in clinical encounters.[8] This dual analogy of clinical detective and interpreter of "texts" and "documents" is based on the parallel assumption that these multiple sets of activities (detecting and interpreting) use everyday, practical knowledge about social structures, typical behaviors, and patterns of interpretation in clinical environments. These activities also exemplify Schutz's insight that the work of identifying the meanings of those structures, behaviors, and patterns, their presuppositions, their languages, their usage, and so on, directly correlates to the specific kind of attention directed to the circumstances (Schutz 1967a; Schutz and Luckman 1973). Thus, the documentary method, with its embrace of disciplined discovery and self-conscious interpretation, emphasizes – even insists – that one follow the questions threaded and woven across events to trace the senses of meaning evoked in clinical circumstances.

Indeed, our readers will notice that this same idea is used to thread and tie the different sections of this book together. Interpretations in the chapters that follow the Zadeh Scenario illustrate important elements regarding what is often taken for granted in actual consultations as well as bring into highlight the contributors' own documentary style, because their interpretations employ both personally and professionally derived everyday knowledge about social structures, roles and relationships, typical behaviors, patterns of interpretation, legitimate vocabularies, and communication styles in clinical as well as more extensive healthcare environments. By highlighting these implications among different levels of inquiry, the aim is to offer our readers a means to trace the style and content of interpretations used by our contributors in order to raise questions and, likewise, to link, correlate, and contrast the themes presented in different sections of the book. Used this way, the documentary method of interpretation can be focused to raise more explicitly the considerations about discernment and delineation of issues and problems at different levels of clinical engagement, including critical assessment about writing about clinical cases and clinical ethics consultation.

---

[8] In *Ethics and the Clinical Encounter* (Zaner 1988/2002), Zaner elaborates to say, "The 'detective work' or 'circumstantial understanding' is an expanded form of the 'documentary method of interpretation,' a methodical rendering of the central concept of *context* [which he had explored in depth in Zaner 1981] and its moral equivalent, *enablement* or empowering" (285). In *Troubled Voices: Stories of Ethics and Illness* (Zaner 1993) he puts it this way: "ethicists help pick out key decision points and options. They help people go through their options and possible outcomes in the light of their own concerns and values, finding what seems most reasonable to them. As the meaning of obscure texts rarely jumps out and announces itself to the reader, the ethicist needs to become a sort of detective, collecting and probing clues and hints" (151).

Organization of the Book

The book is composed of 6 sections, the first of which is this Introduction. Next comes Part One, which is the Zadeh Scenario. Part Two then consists of 5 chapters which present critical reviews of Finder's participation as an ethics consultant as presented in the Zadeh Scenario. Part Three consists of 4 chapters which comment and critically reflect on the Zadeh Scenario as well as the issues raised and methods used in Part Two. Part Four presents 3 chapters which each review the implications for peer review raised by their interrogation of the questions generated by the initial 5 critical reviews of Finder's participation in the ethics consultation presented in the Scenario and combine that review with assessment and critical evaluations of the commentaries about method gathered from the four chapters in Part Three. The final section, Part Five, is a reflective summary and response to several of the more significant considerations raised by the commentaries followed by a more general summary of implications for clinical ethics practice that emerge from this entire effort, i.e., from the Zadeh Project itself.

Our premise for organizing the book in this format is fairly straightforward, although not simple. For each Part, the themes developed in each essay represent a specific approach to the same text – the Zadeh Scenario. We asked each contributor to address his or her own understanding of the conceptual and practical commitments prompted by reading this Scenario, and to write a chapter which reflected those issues they thought merited careful discussion. As the book progresses through each succeeding Part, the authors, by reflecting on all the preceding essays, were tasked with identifying, assessing, and responding to the cumulative increase in the complexity and layering of issues, questions, and methods. These themes, issues, topics, and even lists developed and interrogated by our colleagues serve to demonstrate the multiple perspectives that can be focused on a specific, and fragmentary, expression about everyday clinical ethics encounters. As a key result of this design, the thematic variations among different contributions can be explicated as a means to further identify and emphasize which among all those themes, issues, topics, and so on warrant additional explanation and critical interrogation. Akin to how conversations unfold – and more significantly, in ways analogous to involvement in actual ethics consultation situations – the rewards for this effort are stimulating, intriguing, complex, and relevant.

The Zadeh Scenario: An Unaltered Fragment

As noted, we submitted the Zadeh Scenario to each of our collaborators – in the same manuscript form found (sans typos) within this volume – for those conference sessions we conducted, and likewise to each of the contributors to this volume. However, it must be explicitly stated again that this manuscript was not written for the sake of engaging in these kinds of shared activities. The motivation, rather, was much more personal and specific: an attempt to capture, perhaps in some coherent way, a variety of moments in the experience of actually doing ethics consultation so as to (hopefully) better inform the author (Finder) about his own practice. It was only after the fact, when the Scenario had been shared (with Bliton) that the idea began to emerge that sharing it more broadly might serve as a device through which to learn with others, not merely what they might identify as significant in what Finder did (or did not do) but how, in that process of review, the commitments these collaborators see as important for themselves in their own practices could also be shared.

Because it was not intended to be a full and complete rendering of all that a clinical ethics consultant does while conducting ethics consultation, the Zadeh Scenario presents a "problem," in that is does not exhibit several elements typically assumed for published "ethics cases." Accordingly, this Scenario must be understood, quite plainly, as a fragment. The Scenario nevertheless does pose questions about where, or how, it does, or could, fit into a more complete story.

In that way, although the Zadeh Scenario is not an "ethics case" in the typical way that "ethics cases" are published, there are surely implications which are treated that way by our contributors. Perhaps we should say that instead of representing a "case," this Scenario, as a fragment, is unfinished. This characteristic itself presents crucial implications regarding the sets of assumptions and relevant features now "documented" by the critical inquiries presented in the essays that follow. As Lisa Rasmussen proposes in her essay, the Scenario presents a "lens of a case narrative that is necessarily limited (because it is a distillation of an experience lived through days and weeks of interaction with many people)" (Rasmussen 2018: 151). Indeed, that limitation sets up the range of interpretations generated in the different sections and throughout this volume. For example, Tarris Rosell and Brit Johnson ask at the beginning of their essay a question fundamental to the Project: "Was this an "ethics consultation," or something else entirely? Perhaps it began as an ethics consultation and became something else, or began as something else and became an ethics consultation" (Rosell and Johnson 2018: 99–100). Each reader of the Scenario begins by encountering that question in her/his own way, and hence, from the beginning, it has provided a stable document through which to explore a variety of presumptions and commitments regarding what ethics consultation is, what characteristics delineate "good" clinical ethics practice, which questions demand a response, and so on.

In that light, additional clear questions can be anticipated, and demand emphasis: is writing, or "writing-up," a clinical ethics case consultation presumed to be a kind of clinical report, as it were, a "telling" of the "facts" about "what actually occurred" – where 'actually' is presumed to carry with it the sense of a description of what really and truly happened, and hence what is to be taken as most important? (Zaner 2015: 162–3). If so, how should all of the details that are provided in Finder's telling be conveyed?[9]

---

[9] Tod Chambers and others have argued that writings in bioethics, and more specifically writing about cases in clinical ethics, have their own set of literary devices and rhetorical appeals which,

As we emphasized above, one evident characteristic of clinical practice displayed by the Scenario is a kind of primacy for the conversations and interactions an ethics consultant encounters when entering into a patient's and family's life. Another primary question to be addressed regards how, in what ways precisely, does this talking and listening figure into any evaluation regarding practices of ethics consultation in clinical environments? Beyond that, in what ways do or ought such practical, everyday activities of talking and listening figure into the format and content in the variety of other forms of written documentation, such as the ethics consultant's personal notes, chart notes, case presentations, and so on, as well as writings intended as a critical or interpretive commentary on a specific situation, topic, or theme for professional presentation and publication?

Certainly, Finder was motivated to write this Scenario – and to continue the effort to compose it once he started – by a kind of "hopefulness" that he might learn something about his own practice. And evident in that hopefulness are clear presumptions, not the least of which is that there was *something* going on in the conversations and interactions he had in the course of this consultation that was worth trying to identify and then reflect upon. In that way, the Zadeh Scenario – both in the moments of being written and when that writing was finally "completed" – is open, not merely in the sense of it being a fragment and hence "unfinished" or "unpolished," but also open in the sense of being open to interpretation. Said more simply, the Zadeh Scenario was written as a way to discover something regarding the conduct of ethics consultation – but what that "something" is was not pre-configured, not pre-established, not pre-determined. Accordingly, as stated above, the Scenario was, and continues to be, open to and available for interpretation.

As a fragment, the Zadeh Scenario therefore allows for another sort of openness in its own implication of the larger narratives that did occur and can be imagined – although these are not described or documented in the Scenario. Anticipating the typical possibilities which might have occurred, our commentators make great use of this opportunity to imagine. Again, we are exceedingly grateful for their curiosity and persistence as we worked through the different stages in the development for this Project.

With all of that said, the Zadeh Scenario is published here as a whole fragment and presented with a priority of place at the beginning of the book. As the unaltered touchstone for each essay, it functions as the primary source of themes and thus orients the essays that follow and refer to it. This priority and function in the design of the Zadeh Project create the specific context where the Scenario evokes for our collaborators in this project a set of questions and the need for careful interpretation analogous to those questions and insistent needs that characterize the kind of conversations and inquiries that occur in clinical encounters that involve clinical ethics consultants.

---

having developed within an amalgamation of historical and linguistic practices and genres, may obscure other relevant issues due to the limitations within one or another of worldviews actually involved. See especially Chambers 1994, 1996; Crigger 1995.

Precisely in that context, we need to be explicit about the function of the Zadeh Scenario in that analogy. The analogy we are using has several different elements. The first is that ethical issues in clinical situations are complex – due to the many conceptual and practical commitments embedded in the languages, attitudes, historical and social conventions specific to clinical life. The second is that the "normal way of life" in clinical work is far less stable and guaranteed than it often appears. Indeed, one hallmark of clinical ethics work is its demand (even though not heeded as often as it should be) specifically not to take for granted what is otherwise taken for granted in daily institutional life.

It is that second element which creates an identifiable and crucial component of the complex analogy presented to the individuals invited to contribute to the Zadeh Project. Not only does this story of the Zadeh Scenario illustrate the need for careful appreciation of the unique and particular ways by which the "typical" and "routine" continually result in interactions and outcomes that cannot be predicted, or that confound and go awry – so much so, indeed, that there develop typical ways to deal with the "atypical"[10] – but it also does not present a "case" in a written format typical for "case presentations." In other words, presented in the ordinary everydayness that Finder describes, the Zadeh Scenario solicits from our contributors – again, analogous to the ways that people in clinical situations continually trace out and revise the context and meaning of what they are going through – that specific need for careful appreciation and appraisal of morally relevant features along a considerable range of possibilities.

In that evocative and imaginative way, and emerging directly out of a mosaic of intersections among many different and multiple discourses that compose the field of clinical ethics consultation,[11] the essays that follow after the Zadeh Scenario in Part Two, Part Three, and Part Four contribute a set of rich and lucid discussions that raise sharp questions in response to the ongoing call and clamor about the need for standardized procedures, criteria, and initiatives to credential individual ethics consultants and to certify a range of qualifications.[12] Far from its original, personal, and possibly idiosyncratic origin, the Zadeh Scenario is presented here, as it was presented to our various collaborators beginning with those who participated with us in 2010 for that first panel, with an aim of using and illustrating this documentary

---

[10] Alfred Schutz and Thomas Luckman note that "what is taken for granted does not form a closed, unequivocally articulated and clearly arranged province." Instead, any situation "is surrounded by uncertainty." Also, what is considered typical are typifications prominent in the stock of knowledge that "presents solutions to problems of my previous experiences and acts" (Schutz and Luckman 1973: 9).

[11] We can include here, as examples of such multiple discourses, the discussions about expertise, the standing of moral theories for what is called "practical ethics," as well as discussions regarding the influence of those contentious discourses in the history and development in the field of clinical ethics. See in particular Scofield 2008; Bishop, Fanning, and Bliton 2010; Engelhardt 2012; Callahan 2015.

[12] For instance, the credentialing and certification effort of the ASBH Quality Attestation initiative, as discussed in Kodish et al. 2013, garnered a lot of attention – and critique, which critique continues, as displayed in several of the contributions to this book.

method to discover more about what matters and what may be at stake in the actual practice and growing field of clinical ethics consultation.

An Enduring Theme: Voices, Talking and Listening

No surprise to us, our invitation to our colleagues to critically engage the Zadeh Scenario resulted in the numerous voices and multiple, complex perspectives that readers will encounter in Parts Two, Three, and Four. Their responses reveal much about the diverse standpoints in this field, and plainly show the way these standpoints can and do influence understandings about ethics consultation, clinical practice, and writing about both.

In any development of peer review and credentialing for ethics consultants, considerations about precisely this sort of diversity and complexity will need to be explicitly addressed. As we mentioned earlier, within the design for this Project is a commitment to probe the idea that there are unmistakable needs to accurately interpret, understand, and tell about the different voices that occur in clinical encounters. These needs require explicit moral attention, because, as Zaner has discussed, "among the other voices choired within any encounter one can readily discern the reverberation of moral feelings embodied in images, noises, and gestures, expressed in personal and social discourses – and the urgencies to be heard, even merely noticed" (Zaner 2015: 114). It is these specific activities of interpreting, understanding, and telling in clinical circumstances that provide the most immediate kind of disclosure of individuals as they interact. "For in these encounters," Zaner says elsewhere, "the whole point is that unique individuals are caught up with one another – whether as patients, families, or providers – and to say what that means, what each experiences, and the like, can only mean 'to tell the story'" (Zaner 2010: 274).

The theoretical and practical dimensions of clinical ethics consultation are wide-ranging and complex. As mentioned earlier in this Introduction, a theme prominent for the Zadeh Project is that the clinical and moral work of ethics consultation is primarily communicative, involving many varied forms of listening and telling, and so it is to those communicative dimensions that we must pay careful attention. Clinical ethics consultation, as a practice, is defined and determined by the actual circumstances encountered – a proposal consonant with what Schutz advocated as a principle of method for any serious and rigorous approach to human situations (Schutz 1967b; Schutz and Luckman 1989). This method allows the necessary access to the professional circumstances and sociality of many different and heterogeneous moral stories and claims about moral life. In the concluding chapter we will take up several concerns of this sort about moral stories and claims about moral life in the practice of clinical ethics consultation and the endeavor of peer review and peer learning.

These considerations all contribute to the ongoing work of identifying and probing those experiential and normative positions presented in the multiple arenas of health care, including the set of considerations about human needs and the demands of a shared moral life which emphasizes both understanding and incorporating a plurality of values. After all, although it remains true that every ethical view makes demands on our lives, our actions, and our own commitments, it may well turn out that there is no one correct sort of moral approach, or ethics for that matter; in fact, there very well may be many different options through which to possibly resolve morally complex circumstances (Finder and Bliton 2008). As a result, one realm of clinical ethics directs its attention to inquiring about and pursuing ways that we might understand and incorporate such a plurality of values, and thus live together among our differences. Another realm, as it begins to come into focus, insistently shows our need to fashion and identify those institutions that will support this end.

For example, in addition to using their own professionally derived knowledge and typified understanding of both clinical situations and written commentary about clinical ethics, each of our contributors has his or her own way to interpret the role of ethics consultation in the social environment in which she or he practices, as well as the status for that role in the organization and clinical environments where she or he works. Likewise, within their specific contexts, each has her or his own way to encounter, interpret, and understand what it is like to undergo the hardship of severe moral disquiet, or to be confronted with the sharp and even ultimate issues of human life – such as those that confront the family in the Zadeh Scenario: the experience of a loved one's chronic disease, issues of loss, the limitations of contemporary medical practices to alter these, and the undergoing of rage and guilt and grief. On the basis of his or her own practical experience, each engages in that characteristic activity of focusing and thinking about the efforts and actions specific to his or her own clinical practice of ethics consultation, as well as those moral experiences undergone in that practice. Hence, a defining feature that makes this "clinical" is that this type of reflective vigilance or attentiveness is not merely required, but furthermore the degree of rigor exercised in its inherent "intention" shifts the focal concern (Zaner 1975).

In more straightforward terms, this "intention" characterizes the sustained focus and rigor for a kind of clinical ethics detective work. Consider this kind of shift in intentional focus when it becomes personal, as one collected group of ethicists has explained regarding this exact point: when it is you or your loved one who becomes the patient confronted "face to face with mortality, loss of control, vulnerability and increased dependence," it turns out to be quite a different experience (Dresser 2011: 14). When it is you or your loved one, they insist, we become more alert to "the ethical significance of what some might regard as trivial elements of patient care" (Dresser 2011: 15). In this light, one participant observed that "doctors and nurses make 'constant small ethical decisions [in their] everyday clinical work,' like whether to make eye contact with the patient or take seriously the patient's complaints" (Dresser 2011: 15). In other words, another said, "Without a good understanding of what it is like to be overwhelmed by the experience of illness—one's own or that of a loved one—how can the doctor or ethicist appreciate the human situation the doctor must address?" (Dresser 2011: 17).

In a similar way, our contributors "document" in their writing these pivotal elements of focusing and thinking about the efforts and actions specific to clinical ethics consultation. Incorporated in their "documentation" are those specific sets of situations, expectations, norms and so on, that each has encountered, interpreted, and then utilized in his or her experience of moral issues, social concerns, and institutional attitudes in clinical work – embedded as all those elements are in their own experiences in clinical routines and practices, along with the specific history and formation of their own professional roles and activities. In summary, their contributions "document" critical ways to understand the broad and extensive array of critical issues and questions regarding what might be at stake in the telling of the Zadeh Scenario, and at the same time, the Scenario also represents simply another set of experiences in a series of everyday occurrences. That is to say, our contributors illustrate the multiple ways that clinical ethics and related matters are understood from their role as peer reviewers and commentators and, likewise, clearly show how the range of interpretations woven throughout these different chapters serve as exemplars for describing the contents not merely of "ethical problems" but also, and perhaps most importantly, what it could mean to "do" clinical ethics consultation.

As we did when initially sending all of our collaborators the invitation to join us in this exploration, we now invite you, the reader, to join us as well in this process of discovery, this effort to be open, this work of giving voice to what might be held as meaningful at the root of clinical ethics practice; this, in short, is the ultimate aim of the Zadeh Project.

References

Andre J (2002) Bioethics as practice. University of North Carolina Press, Chapel Hill

Anspach R (1995) Deciding who lives: fateful choices in the intensive-care nursery. University of California Press, Oakland

Aulisio MP, Arnold RA, Youngner SJ (2003) Ethics consultation: from theory to practice. John Hopkins University Press, Baltimore

Bishop JP, Fanning JB, Bliton MJ (2010) Echo calling narcissus: what exceeds the gaze of clinical ethics consultation. HEC Forum 22(1):73–85

Bliton MJ (2005) Richard Zaner's "troubled" voice in *Troubled Voices*: poseur, posing, possibilizing? Theor Med Bioeth 26(1):25–53

Bliton MJ, Finder SG (2002) Traversing boundaries: clinical ethics, moral experience, and the withdrawal of life supports. Theor Med Bioeth 23(3):233–258

Bosk CL (2009) What would you do? juggling bioethics and ethnography. University of Chicago Press, Chicago

Bruce CR, Smith ML, Tawose OM, Sharp RR (2014) Practical guidance for charting ethics consultations. HEC Forum 26(1):79–93

Bruce CR, Eves MM, Allen NG et al (2015) "Systematizing" ethics consultations services. HEC Forum 27(1):35–45

Callahan D (2015) What is it to do good ethics? J Med Ethics 41(1):68–70

Chambers TS (1994) The bioethicist as author: the medical ethics case as rhetorical device. Lit Med 13(1):60–78

Chambers TS (1996) From the ethicist's point of view: the literary nature of ethical inquiry. Hastings Cent Rep 26(1):25–33

Chambers TS (2000) Why ethicists should stop writing cases. J Clin Ethics 11(3):206–218

Churchill LR, Fanning JB, Schenk D (2013) What patients teach: the everyday ethics of health care. Oxford University Press, New York
Crigger BJ (1995) Negotiating the moral order: paradoxes of ethics consultation. Kennedy Inst Ethics J 5(2):89–112
Curtis JR, Engelberg RA, Bensink ME et al (2012) End-of-life care in the intensive care unit: can we simultaneously increase quality and reduce costs? Am J Respir Crit Care Med 186(7):587–592
Dresser R (2011) Bioethics and cancer: when the professional becomes personal. Hastings Cent Rep 41(6):14–18
Dubler NN, Webber MP, Swiderski DM et al (2009) Charting the future: credentialing, privileging, quality, and evaluation in clinical ethics consultation. Hastings Cent Rep 39(6):23–33
Engelhardt HT (1996) The foundations of bioethics, 2nd edn. Oxford University Press, New York
Engelhardt HT (2012) A skeptical reassessment of bioethics. In: Engelhardt HT (ed) Bioethics critically reconsidered. Philosophy and medicine 100. Springer, New York, pp 1–30
Evans JH (2012) The history and future of bioethics: a sociological view. Oxford University Press, New York
Finder SG (2018) The Zadeh scenario. In: Finder SG, Bliton MJ (eds) Peer review, peer education, and modeling in the practice of clinical ethics consultation: the Zadeh project. Springer, Cham, pp 21–42
Finder SG, Bliton MJ (2008) Responsibility in actual practice: consent and participation in clinical ethics consultation. In: Hester M (ed) Ethics by committee: a textbook on consultation, organization, and education. Rowman & Littlefield, Lantham, pp 79–106
Finder SG, Bliton MJ (2011) Responsibility after the apparent end: "following-up" in clinical ethics consultation. Bioethics 25(7):413–424
Fins JJ, Kodish E, Cohn F et al (2016) A pilot evaluation of portfolios for quality attestation of clinical ethics consultants. AJOB 16(3):15–24
Foglia MB, Fox E, Chanko B, Bottrell MM (2012) Preventive ethics: addressing ethics quality gaps on a systems level. Jt Comm J Qual Patient Saf 38(3):103–111
Ford PJ, Dudzinski DM (eds) (2008) Complex ethics consultations: cases that haunt us. Cambridge University Press, Cambridge
Fox RC, Swazey JP (2008) Observing Bioethics. Oxford University Press, New York
Frank AW (1997) Illness as moral occasion: restoring agency to ill people. Health Interdiscip J Soc Study Health Illn Med 1(2):131–148
Frank AW (2001) Experiencing illness through storytelling. In: Kay Toombs S (ed) Handbook of phenomenology and medicine. Philosophy and medicine series, vol 68. Kluwer Academic Publishers, Dordrecht, pp 229–246
Frank AW (2004) Ethics as process and practice. Intern Med J 34(6):355–357
Freedman B, Weijer C, Brereza E (1993) Case notes and charting of bioethics case consultations. HEC Forum 5(3):176–195
Gaines AD, Juengst ET (2008) Origin myths in bioethics: constructing sources, motives and reason in bioethic(s). Cult Med Psychiatry 32(3):303–327
Garfinkel H (1967) Studies in ethnomethodology. Prentice-Hall, Inc., Englewood Cliffs
Hoffmaster B (1992) Can ethnography save the life of medical ethics? Soc Sci Med 35(12):1421–1431
Jecker NS, Jonsen AR, Pearlman RA (eds) (2012) Bioethics: an introduction to the history, methods and practice, 3rd edn. Jones & Bartlett, Sudbury
Jonsen AR, Toulmin S (1988) The abuse of casuistry: a history of moral reasoning. University of California Press, Los Angeles
Kaufman S (2015) Ordinary medicine: extraordinary treatments, longer lives, and where to draw the line. Duke University Press, Durham
Kleinman A (1988) The illness narratives: suffering, healing, and the human condition. Basic Books, New York
Kleinman A (2006) What really matters: living a moral life amidst danger and uncertainty. Oxford University Press, Oxford

Kodish E, Fins JJ, Braddock C et al (2013) Quality attestation for clinical ethics consultants: a two-step model from the American society for bioethics and humanities. Hastings Cent Rep 43(5):26–36

Komesaroff P (2001) The many faces of the clinic: a Levinasian view. In: Kay Toombs S (ed) Handbook of phenomenology and medicine. Philosophy and medicine series, vol 68. Kluwer Academic Publishers, Dordrecht, pp 317–330

MacIntyre A (1984) After virtue, 2nd edn. University of Notre Dame Press, Notre Dame

Molewijk B, Kleinlugtenbeit D, Pugh SM et al (2011) Emotions and clinical ethics support: a moral inquiry into emotions in moral case deliberation. HEC Forum 23(4):257–268

Molewijk B, Widdershoven G, Vollman J, Schildmann J (2016) What quality is actually assessed within written records? AJOB 16(3):48–50

Natanson M (1970) The journeying self: a study in philosophy and social role. Addison-Wesley Publishing Co., Reading

Nelson WA, Gardent PB, Shulman E, Splaine ME (2010) Preventing ethics conflicts and improving healthcare quality through system redesign. Qual Safe Health Care 19:526–530

Pearlman R, Foglia MB, Fox E et al (2016) Ethics consultation quality assessment tool: a novel method for assessing the quality of ethics case consultations based on written records. AJOB 16(3):3–14

Rasmussen L (2018) Standardizing the case narrative. In: Finder SG, Bliton MJ (eds) Peer review, peer education, and modeling in the practice of clinical ethics consultation: the Zadeh project. Springer, Cham, pp 151–160

Rogers MF (1983) Sociology, ethnomethodology, and experience: a phenomenological critique. Cambridge University Press, London

Rosell T, Johnson B (2018) This may, or may not, be an ethics consultation. In: Finder SG, Bliton MJ (eds) Peer review, peer education, and modeling in the practice of clinical ethics consultation: the Zadeh project. Springer, Cham, pp 99–107

Schutz A (1967a) The phenomenology of the social world (trans: Walsh G, Walsh FLG). Evanston: Northwestern University Press

Schutz A (1967b) Sartre's theory of the alter ego. In: Natanson M (ed) Collected papers I: the problem of social reality, 2nd unchanged edn. Martinus Nijhoff, The Hague, pp 180–203

Schutz A, Luckman T (1973) Structures of the life-world, vol I (trans: Zaner RM, Engelhardt HT). Evanston: Northwestern University Press

Schutz A, Luckman T (1989) The structures of the life-world, vol II (trans: Zaner RM, Parent DJ). Evanston: Northwestern University Press

Scofield GR (2008) What is medical ethics consultation? J Law Med Ethics 36(1):95–118

Speigelberg H (1975) Doing phenomenology: essays on and in phenomenology. Martinus Nijoff, The Hague, pp 68–69

Starr P (1982) The social transformation of American medicine: the rise of a sovereign profession and the making of a vast industry. Basic Books, New York

Zaner RM (1975) On the sense of method in phenomenology. In: Pivcevic E (ed) Phenomenology and philosophical understanding. Cambridge University Press, London, pp 125–141

Zaner RM (1981) The context of self: a phenomenological inquiry using medicine as a Clue. Ohio University Press, Athens

Zaner RM (1984) Is "ethicist" anything to call a philosopher? Hum Stud 7(1):71–90

Zaner RM (1988) Ethics and the clinical encounter. Prentice-Hall, Inc., Englewood Cliffs (reprinted in 2002 by Academic Renewal Press)

Zaner RM (1993) Troubled voices: stories of ethics and illness. The Pilgrim Press, Cleveland

Zaner RM (1998) In response: what's it *really* all about? Hum Stud 21(1):63–70

Zaner RM (2004a) Conversations on the edge. Georgetown University Press, Washington, DC

Zaner RM (2004b) Physicians and patients in relation: clinical interpretation and dialogues of trust. In: Khushf G (ed) Handbook of bioethics: taking stock of the field from a philosophical perspective. Kluwer Academic Publishers, Dordrecht/Boston, pp 223–250

Zaner RM (2006) The phenomenon of vulnerability in clinical encounters. Hum Stud 29(3):283–294
Zaner RM (2010) A phenomenological reflection conducted through narrative: an essay in honor of Lester Embree. In: Nenon T, Blosse P (eds) Advancing phenomenology: essays in honor of Lester Embree. Springer, New York, pp 271–301
Zaner RM (2015) A critical examination of ethics in health care and biomedical research: voices and vision. Springer, New York
Zussman R (1992) Intensive care: medical ethics and the medical profession. University of Chicago Press, Chicago

PART ONE
A CLINICAL ETHICS CONSULTATION NARRATIVE

The Zadeh Scenario

Stuart G. Finder

A First Encounter

> "I beg of you, Doctor, please don't let Dr. Moore see my mother again. My sisters and I do not want him talking with us anymore."

So concluded my first conversation with Samir Zadeh. Our meeting had been purely accidental; as I walked onto the elevator going down from the Surgical ICU, he and one of his sisters (her name, I would learn, was Nadira) were already on, coming down from another one of our hospital's ICUs, from a floor above. Samir was a man in his early 50s, and his sister, whom I would learn was actually a few years older, appeared younger than he. They were talking quietly when the doors opened, but as is often the case in elevators, especially in a hospital, as soon as I entered, their conversation stopped. We rode down to the bottom floor in silence. As we exited, I let them go first, a courtesy I had been taught by my parents, and they both thanked me, in the usual social way, and walked out into the lobby and then out of the building. I walked the same way.

It was when we were about 25 feet from the building that Mr. Zadeh and his sister stopped, so that I caught up to them. As I did, Mr. Zadeh, a large man, maybe 6 feet tall and 250 pounds, with thinning hair and a well-groomed mustache, turned and said my name aloud, "Dr. Finder, may you be so kind as to talk?"

"Uh, sure," I replied. "Have we met?"

This scenario is based on an actual clinical ethics consultation. Various details were altered upon its writing, including names, gender, age and other identifiers, in order to protect the confidentiality of all participants other than the author.

S. G. Finder (✉)
Center for Healthcare Ethics, Cedars-Sinai Medical Center, Los Angeles, CA, USA
e-mail: Stuart.Finder@cshs.org

S. G. Finder, M. J. Bliton (eds.), *Peer Review, Peer Education, and Modeling in the Practice of Clinical Ethics Consultation: The Zadeh Project*,
https://doi.org/10.1007/978-3-319-90955-4_2

It was a reflex to ask him that because in that split second of his turning and saying my name, I was also a bit taken off guard and wondered how he knew who I was. After all, other than having seen him on the elevator, I couldn't recall having previously met him.

"No, and my apology for being so abrupt. But I saw on your name badge that you are the Director of Ethics and so I was thinking, Dr. Moore, he might work under you?"

Steve Moore is one of my colleagues.

"Well, yes. Dr. Moore is my colleague. How do you know him?"

And with that, Mr. Zadeh began to tell me about his mother who was a patient in one of our ICUs. A woman of 83, she had been diagnosed with lung cancer 3 years ago, but while other physicians had recommended she pursue hospice ("Those doctors she saw, they told her her cancer was an aggressive kind and already had spread too far," he stated), Mr. Zadeh and his sisters (Nadira, who was the woman with Mr. Zadeh and whom he introduced to me, although she mostly just stood by quietly while her brother spoke, and Farzana, the oldest who, he said, was currently up with her mother) found an oncologist (Dr. Said Broukhim) who was willing to pursue aggressive treatments. "And," Nadira interjected, "he has given our mother three extra years."

Mr. Zadeh continued that his mother had done well and even though she'd been sick, she had continued to take care of his father—her husband—who had dementia and had been in decline for years (I would learn later that several months ago he'd been hospitalized and then gone to rehab, from which he was scheduled to be discharged soon. In addition to helping take care of their mother, Mr. Zadeh and his sisters had also been dealing with their father's illness).

"Two weeks ago," Mr. Zadeh now said, "I stopped by to see my mother, and as soon as I entered her home I knew something was not right. And I found her in her bed, confused and not able to speak. I tell you, Dr. Finder, I was very afraid, to see my mother like this. So I called 911 and they sent an ambulance and we came to your hospital and my mother was admitted."

As Mr. Zadeh was relaying this to me, I began to remember Steve telling me about Mrs. Hamadani (whose last name, it turned out, was different from her son's). Steve had initially seen her back when she was first in the hospital 3 years ago, even before Dr. Broukhim became her oncologist. At that time, her neurologist, who had been following her because of her having Parkinson's, had requested ethics consultation because he believed the family's request for aggressive intervention for her then newly diagnosed cancer was inappropriate; beyond her Parkinson's and the mets to her liver and brain, she also suffered from CHF and renal insufficiency, if I was remembering correctly. But I did remember that Steve had said that this neurologist was the one who had suggested hospice, and that Mr. Zadeh and his sisters had vilified him, actually shouting him out of their mother's room and yelling down the hall that he was fired. It had been quite a scene from what Steve had learned and later told me, and several of the nurses had actually contemplated calling security. The Neurologist, though, unfazed, simply called us and asked for an ethics consultation, and Steve had picked it up. In an effort to help this family, Steve was the one who had actually contacted Dr. Broukhim to see if he'd be willing to talk with Mr. Zadeh and his sisters. Broukhim had a reputation of being extremely aggressive—often too much so for some of the others physicians who frequently interacted with him—but he was beloved by his patients.

And while Mr. Zadeh did not mention it to me now, I knew his mother had been in and out of the hospital five times over the past 3 years. I knew this because each time she came in, she would pop up on our list (one of the benefits of an electronic medical record is that you can keep track of when patients with whom you've been involved return to the hospital) and Steve would stop by and check in with her and her children. More importantly, Steve and I had talked about what had happened on several of those admissions, had even used it as an example in one of our Clinical Ethics Consultation Service Review sessions, namely, someone involved in her care—perhaps the consulting nephrologists or the ICU attending or the Social Worker—would informally ask Steve, when they saw that he was checking in on Mrs. Hamadani, to more formally intervene because they were concerned that Mrs. Hamadani was suffering, that continued intervention was futile, that her children were making bad decisions. And Steve would then talk to the various physicians involved, including Dr. Broukhim, in order to learn if there was a shared opinion about the possible inappropriateness of Mrs. Hamadani's treatment plan, but there never was. Moreover, no one was willing to take the lead and more officially state, in Mrs. Hamadani's medical record or at a family care conference, that continued treatment would not be appropriate, should not be pursued. So Steve simply followed along.

Then, 2 weeks ago, when Mrs. Hamadani was admitted, Dr. Broukhim had immediately called Steve and asked for his help; he now felt there was nothing more he could do, that Mrs. Hamadani was at the end. He thus wanted Steve to help him talk with Mrs. Hamadani's children. Broukhim also requested Palliative Care get involved and he sought input from Nephrology, Cardiology, and Neurology. I remembered Steve telling me that this may have been a first with Broukhim!

Within 2 days, all of the physicians involved in Mrs. Hamadani's care had left notes in her chart stating that further aggressive intervention was not warranted, and that DNAR status would be appropriate. With this in hand, Dr. Broukhim had asked Steve to join him in meeting with the family.

During this family meeting, which Steve had told me about and which was held on the third day of Mrs. Hamadani's hospitalization, Dr. Broukhim had been exceptionally clear and direct that he believed that Mrs. Hamadani was not only no longer a candidate for chemotherapy, but, for that matter, any curative intervention, that she was at the end of her life and that the best thing to do now was to keep her comfortable. Indeed, to Steve's chagrin—because it wasn't really accurate—Dr. Broukhim even said that Mrs. Hamadani's condition was such that some would claim that under the hospital's "medically inappropriate treatment" policy, to do otherwise could not be justified.

Mrs. Hamadani's son and daughters were, Steve had told me, quite distressed by Dr. Broukhim's report, especially this man with whom I was now conversing. And yet they expressed great appreciation for Dr. Broukhim and all that he had done to help their mother. At first Steve thought that they were ready to accept Broukhim's recommendation to shift purely to a comfort only focus. But then, when the issue of code status was raised by Steve as a practical example of what it means to focus on comfort only, they were adamant that they were not ready to make that kind of decision. Moreover, they wanted a G-tube placed because they believed that with more aggressive nutritional intervention, their mother would be able to rally. When Dr. Broukhim told them that the extent of her disease was such that she was not a candidate for any type of surgery, and thus that a G-tube could not be safely placed, Mr. Zadeh asked that an NG tube be placed instead.

Interestingly, as I began to remember these details, Mr. Zadeh also began to tell me his version of that initial meeting with Steve, and then the subsequent two-plus weeks of his mother's hospitalization. As I listened, I continued to remember what Steve had told me.

Specifically, at this point in that conversation on the third day of Mrs. Hamadani's hospitalization, the tension in the room had been palpable, both in terms of Mrs. Hamadani's children being agitated by the prospect of some sort of final decision being made not to provide additional interventions for their mother, and Dr. Broukhim being agitated by having the children ask him for more interventions and him having to say "no," an unusual experience for him. In an effort to help defuse the moment, Steve had offered that perhaps it would not be unreasonable to place the NG, since it offered little risk and only minimal discomfort given Mrs. Hamadani's state. But Steve also stated that he would like to know what Mr. Zadeh and his sisters were thinking such that they seemeed to be willing to proceed with aggressive intervention given Dr. Broukhim's—and the other physicians' as well—recommendations and concerns.

This gamble, so to speak, paid off in that Mr. Zadeh expressed appreciation to Steve for supporting their wishes for the NG while at the same time acknowledging that his question was a good one, that they really did need to give it more thought, and that they would. In the meantime, however, they still wanted their mother to be full code, and if necessary, to be transferred to the ICU. And as it turned out, several hours after the meeting, Dr. Broukhim did decide that with continued hypotension and respiratory distress, Mrs. Hamadani needed to be transferred to the ICU.

When Steve next stopped by to talk with Mr. Zadeh and his sisters a few days later, they were, he told me, more distressed than they had been during the family meeting. Still, Steve had asked them about the question with which he had left them and if they had come up with an answer yet. I also knew from Steve that while he had stopped by several more times in order to address this, each time Mr. Zadeh or one of his sisters had stated something to the effect, "now is not a good time to talk."

Now, as I stood outside in the plaza, beyond the front doors of the hospital, Mr. Zadeh was telling me what had transpired since what I already knew had occurred, and more specifically, what had occurred not more than an hour or so earlier today.

"My mother, she is strong and after only a few days in the ICU she was well enough to go back to the floor. But the nurses there, they were not as attentive as the staff in the ICU, and my sister, Nadira, or our older sister, Farzana, or I would have to make sure they gave her medicines on time and that they fed her correctly. Let me tell you Dr. Finder, we had to watch out or she would not get the care she needs to get stronger."

As he spoke, Mr. Zadeh was becoming more impassioned, and yet his tone was modulated; it was mostly his gestures and facial expressions that suggested to me that he was more engaged.

"Dr. Broukhim is such a caring man, we are so grateful to him. Unlike those other physicians who didn't want to take care of our mother when she first became sick, he knew that she still had more time to be with us on this earth. And even as my mother has gotten sicker, he still has shown us hope. And he would come and visit, even in the middle of the night. My sisters and I take turns staying with my mother, and sometimes it would be 2:00 in the morning and in would come Dr. Brouhkim, to check on our mother."

"But Dr. Finder," Mr. Zadeh continued, "your Dr. Moore, he has pestered us, always showing up when my mother has come into the hospital, asking us if we are ready to stop. It's as if he doesn't know what it means to love your mother." Mr. Zadeh's voice now began to rise and even quiver slightly. "And then today, my mother was not doing so well, and it is, I believe, because they have not been giving her enough nutrition and so she is weak. And she began to have difficulty breathing and she had to be emergently taken back to the ICU. You look like a gentle man, Dr. Finder, and so I believe you can imagine the worry this caused for us."

Mr. Zadeh's sister, Nadira, was gently wiping her eyes as Mr. Zadeh spoke.

"But what do we find when we come into the ICU but Dr. Moore, standing there and talking with the nurses and doctors. And then the lady ICU doctor asks us to leave our mother's side and to come with her and Dr. Moore into a conference room. Why would they do that when she is having trouble keeping her breath, why would they ask us to leave her side at this time? After all, Dr. Finder, we are not dumb people. We know that our mother has cancer and now she is very sick, so why would we leave her? It makes no sense."

"But the lady doctor was very insistent and Dr. Moore too said that we needed to talk, and so Farzana, as the eldest, and I as the son, we went with Dr. Moore and the ICU doctor, but Nadira stayed with my mother because we could not leave her alone. And when we got into that conference room, I tell you Dr. Finder, I could not believe it. This lady doctor tells us that our mother is at a critical point and that we need to decide if we want her to be placed on the ventilator. But she asked as if it was not our decision, that it was she and Dr. Moore who would decide. And I told them that no decision like that needed to be made until her heart stops; then we, my sisters and I, will decide what to do."

"And then Dr. Moore started to talk about the doctors' belief that she was dying, that her organs are failing and that we needed to make decisions about how she would want to be treated. And so 'why,' I ask, 'why are you having us sit in here instead of being with her as a family?' And this lady doctor just sat there, and Dr. Moore once again started to talk about making decisions before my mother's heart stops, and I said, 'We will tell you what to do when her hearts stop, but until then, we do not want to be sitting here.' I must apologize, Dr. Finder, I was so upset. And poor Farzana was beside herself. Is this anyway to treat someone's mother?"

I was listening intently, trying not only to hear the words but absorb the emotion, the sense of urgency, the experience that this man, whom I had met by accident by stepping onto an elevator, was now offering to me. I made the choice to speak to him.

"I don't think I can really imagine what that was like for you, Mr. Zadeh," I offered, unsure what else to say, unsure whether my decision to speak now was the right thing to do. He took a somewhat deep breath and began to speak again, and so I listened once more.

"And so I asked Dr. Moore, 'Did Frank Sinatra's family have to have these conversations?' It was not a nice thing to say, and I would hope no family would be faced with this kind of thing. And there was Dr. Moore, talking about what we had discussed 2 weeks ago with Dr. Broukhim and how he had come by to visit with us. But he did not *visit*, he simply came to get us to say what he wanted to hear. And it was too much, it was not right, and I again told Dr. Moore and the lady physician that when my mother's heart stop, then we will decide whether to put her on the machines. And then Farzana and I got up and left so that we could be with Nadira and our mother, who, by the way, seems to be doing well with a face mask."

Mr. Zadeh paused, but it was a longer pause than before, as if he was collecting himself, regaining his calm.

"You are a good listener, Dr. Finder, and I thank you. I believe you understand what it is like to face this sort of thing." And then he said it: "And so I beg of you, Doctor, please don't let Dr. Moore see my mother again. My sisters and I do not want him talking with us anymore."

And for a second time since exiting the elevator and walking outside, I was taken aback somewhat. While there was a kind of forcefulness to Mr. Zadeh's request, as he spoke it, both he and his sister Nadira were both looking at me not with anger nor reproach, but with eyes slightly wide and down-turned at the corners. I was struck by their sadness and apprehension, peppered with a bit of fear.

I also was not unaware that I may have just been manipulated.

Moreover, I knew I didn't know what was *really* going on, that the flashes of memory I was having of Mrs. Hamadani's situation were just that, flashes. I couldn't be sure I was remembering accurately and while I had no reason to doubt what Mr. Zadeh had just told me, I also knew that, even if accurate, it was an accurate report of what he had been facing and experiencing; but as always, there was likely much more to the story. And so I wasn't sure it would be the right thing to pull Steve from what was going on even though I don't think it appropriate to force family members to talk with ethics consultants even if we continue to meet with members of the patient care team.

"I will talk with him," I said, "and then I'll come talk with you again too, if that's alright."

"Yes, thank you, Dr. Finder, thank you."

And with that, Mr. Zadeh grabbed my hand with both of his and lightly bowed his head down, and then he and his sister continued walking in the direction they had been going, away from the hospital.

Still taken aback from this whole situation, I was unsure what to do. This was, in many ways, a quite extraordinary conversation. To begin, I had never been stopped like that before, never had a family come up to me out of the blue, in this sort of more public area, and start discussing their situation because they saw "Ethics" on my ID badge. Then there's the fact that one of my colleagues had already been involved such that, even if not immediately, I was able, while in the conversation, to have some recognition about some of what was going on. And then, of course, the most dramatic element, to have the family ask me to intervene on their behalf in order to stop my colleague from talking with them as well as, if I understood correctly, even from checking in on their mother; that too was unprecedented.

I knew I had to talk with Steve, and I was thinking it would also probably be helpful to take a look at Mrs. Hamadani's chart and talk with the ICU staff in order to learn more about what her medical condition looked like today. I also was thinking that it might be useful to talk with Dr. Broukhim. And, I also found myself thinking that I probably needed to find the nearest place to sit down and write out the description of what had just happened. Because I knew well from experience that as soon as I took a next step after this conversation, my recollection of it would change.

And so I chose to walk back to my office, to then sit down and write down a few notes about Mr. Zadeh and his sister Nadira stopping me and talking with me and asking me to intervene. I also was hoping that in doing so, I might provide myself with some time to think more about this conversation I'd just had and to see what might present itself as the right next step to take.

Talking with Steve

After outlining the main elements of my encounter with Mr. Zadeh and his sister, I pulled up Mrs. Hamadani's electronic records and was able to confirm that my recollection of what had been going on with her medically, as well as some of the social dynamics surrounding her care, were as I had thought. I then called Steve.

When I recounted what had happened, he said he was not at all surprised.

"When I've gone to talk with Mr. Zadeh, sometimes he's very nice and even charming, and then I'll see him a few days later and I'm not sure if he's sleep deprived or just really angry, but it's clear he doesn't want to talk with me. So I just say 'Hi,' and leave. And the nurses have told me horror stories, that he and his sisters hover around their mother and are always watching every little thing the nurses do, and if one does something this way but it's not like the last nurse did, which was that way, they get upset. Some of the nurses are even refusing to take care of her anymore because of this. I guess it's been this way every time she comes in."

"And then this afternoon, I was up in the Unit looking into a different situation when I heard the nurses and residents talking about Mrs. Hamadani coming back over. So I started talking with them about what was going on. And then I pulled

Annie Smith aside, since she's attending this week in the Unit, to talk with her, so when they came in and they saw us talking, I'm sure it set them off a bit." And then Steve proceeded to tell me about the meeting, and surprisingly, his recounting was not much different from what Mr. Zadeh had reported, at least in terms of the facts; while the tenor of how Mr. Zadeh had spoken was quite similar to how Mr. Zadeh had presented it to me, Steve's version of his own presentation was not quite as Mr. Zadeh had characterized it.

As for the request that he not be involved, I wasn't surprise at how Steve replied:

"Look, I don't want to make matters worse for this family. I know their coming from a good place, that they want what's best for their mother. They're in a really bad situation and I can only imagine how difficult it must be. As you know, Broukhim is really aggressive and he sometimes gives what I think is false hopes, so I'm not surprised this family is struggling. I'm a bit surprised they saw my coming by to check on them as badgering, and I hope you don't think that's what I was doing…" I assured him I didn't. "I'd just warn you that they may be using you, to avoid what we'd already agreed upon in terms of talking about why they want to code her and have the feeding tube and whatever other aggressive interventions that may be available."

We talked a bit more about the conversations he'd had with Broukhim and the other physicians as well as a bit more about his interactions with Mrs. Hamadani's children. Mostly, Steve told me, he'd been talking with Mr. Zadeh, although one or both of the sisters was always in the room, and he'd spoken with one of them more than the other, although he really didn't know which one it was—"I can't remember their names, but it was the taller one," he said.

I would later learn this was Farzana, the eldest daughter and actually the oldest of the three siblings and the one who'd lived in the United States longest as well.

I knew Steve well enough to know that, at times, even though unintended, he does come across a bit forcefully, with a kind of intensity, because he's really committed to this work and really believes in tying to help, so it wasn't hard for me to imagine that even his simple act of sticking his head into Mrs. Hamadani's room to see if now would be a good time to talk could easily be experienced as invasive. And having heard more about the situation and what Steve and Dr. Broukhim and the nurses had been discussing, I decided that it would be better if Steve stayed clear of the room.

"Of course," I told him, "that doesn't mean you can't be on the Unit if other consults come up. And I think it's OK if you want to keep talking with Broukhim since you've been helping him as much as anything. But really try not to put yourself in a position that the family might mis-perceive as your still being involved with them. I'll take over that. I'm also going to give Broukhim a call since I'm thinking it may be helpful for him and I together to sit down with all three of the kids just to update them on what's going on and to see if they have any questions."

Steve said he was fine with that.

"But I've got to tell you again," he interjected, "be careful. I don't mean this with any disrespect, and I know it sounds bad but, this is a Persian family and they approach these things a lot differently. I've seen it before where they say one thing one day and then the next day it's something different. And especially when it's an elderly parent, they have a really hard time letting go. And it's not just them. You've looked at the chart, you've seen who's involved: Broukhim, Teharani, Nadouri, Hekmat. All these physicians, you know them, and you also well know most of their patients come from their own community, so even if unintentional, there are issues of professional reputation and community standing they have to deal with."

While it could come across not as he intended, I knew Steve was not speaking out of prejudice but out of recognition that as much as anything, cultural elements here may well have been part of what was at play. I also knew we'd be talking more about what was going on with Mrs. Hamadani's situation. I thanked him and hung up.

Based on our conversation and what Steve hold told me he knew of Mrs. Hamadani's current medical condition (although in the ICU, she was stable, and maybe even slightly improved hemodynamically speaking) as well as what I had read in Mrs. Hamadani's electronic record, I didn't feel particularly pressed to do more at this point; after all, it was late in the afternoon. So I decided that come morning I'd call Dr. Broukhim as well as go to the Unit and talk with the folks there.

This was looking to be a very interesting consultation.

A Slight Delay

My plan had been, in the morning, to walk over to the ICU in which Mrs. Hamadani was located, review her paper chart, talk with the ICU team about what was going on, and try to get a hold of Dr. Broukhim. Unfortunately, my role in the institution is not limited to my clinical work, and I was called away for the day due to a number of other situations which, for a variety of reasons, could not wait. Hence, by the time I was done with all of that work, it was already late in the afternoon. I checked the electronic record and saw that medically, Mrs. Hamadani's condition was virtually unchanged from the day before. There being no new Social Work or Case Management notes, I decided once again to wait before going up to the Unit. I did, however, call Dr. Broukhim but only got his voicemail; I left a message letting him know that Steve and I were now both involved and that I wanted to talk with him about what was going on.

Talking with Dr. Brouhkim

After attending a number of pre-scheduled meetings, I finally made my way to the ICU early in the afternoon. Having already done a quick review of her electronic record before going, once in the Unit, as is my usual practice, I grabbed the binder that was Mrs. Hamadani's paper chart and began working my way through what was now nearly 3 weeks of hand-written notes, with an occasional printed electronic note interspersed. I also saw the notes Steve had told me he'd left, both hand-written, from before and then after the meeting at which he had joined Dr. Broukhim in talking with Mrs. Hamadani's children back on the third day of Mrs. Hamadani's hospitalization, as well as his hand-written note from two days prior, the day of the meeting which had led Mr. Zadeh to ask me to remove Steve from the case.

I also saw the various notes Dr. Brouhkim had left, and having yet to hear back from him, I again called his office. One of his Assistants answered and after giving her a quick summary of why I was calling, she patched me through to him. This was actually the first time I had ever spoken with Said Broukhim, although I had known of him for some time. And I knew of his reputation of being extremely aggressive, of even other Oncologists thinking that he pushed the boundaries. But our conversation didn't fit the stereotype.

"Ah, Dr. Finder, I am so sorry not to have called you back sooner. I have been very busy, and with Mrs. Hamadani actually stabilizing over the past 36 hours, I knew we had some time. But I am very glad you have called. I take it you've seen my notes from the past 2 days?"

Indeed, I had. And unlike many others, Said Broukhim still wrote—well, actually, dictated—extensive notes, often 4 or more pages of narrative. He included detail not only of his patients' medical condition, but also the psychosocial dynamics associated with their care. The notes for Mrs. Hamadani gave a very clear picture of all that had been going on, including his own assessment that Mrs. Hamadani was no longer a candidate for any kind of therapeutic interventions, that he had, since the beginning of this admission, been recommending a shift to a purely palliative focus, that the family seemed to understand that their mother was likely near the end of her life, but that they also were, as of yet, unwilling to consent to anything less than full code and that they continued to ask about what other options might be considered. He also referenced Steve's notes and the conversations he and Steve had been having.

Perhaps more extraordinarily, again given his reputation, is that in reference to the meeting Steve and Annie Smith (the "lady doctor" to whom Mr. Zadeh had referred) had had with the family when Mrs. Hamadani had come back into the ICU, Dr. Broukhim explicitly wrote, "I have explained to the patient's family that I had personally asked Dr. Moore to continue to follow the patient closely to try to provide as much support to the family as well as to try to delineate ethical issues involving the care of this terminally ill patient." His note then continued, "I also explained to the patient's family that the reason for ethics evaluation is not to persuade or to be abrasive to the patient's family and it is just to provide more care for them in these trying times."

But I expected the real focus of his question was whether I had seen his note from this morning which detailed a meeting he had had with all three of Mrs. Hamadani's children and which had also been attended by Dr. Smith and Dr. Nadouri, the consulting nephrologist. In that note, a few things stood out.

First, there was the fact that Dr. Broukhim began by mentioning that at the beginning of the session, Mr. Zadeh spoke at some length about his interactions with Steve such that Dr. Brouhkim explicitly wrote that "we did explain to him that this meeting is not about Dr. Moore or Ethics Consultation but only about his mother."

This was then immediately followed by an overview of Drs. Brouhkim, Nadouri, and Smith's assessments of Mrs. Hamadani's status, the real possibility of worsening respirations developing, Dr. Smith's opinion that if she were to be intubated there would be a good chance she'd not be able to be successfully extubated, and her poor renal function. Moreover, he wrote that both he and Dr. Nadouri would not recommend pursuing dialysis if it came to that, their basis being that "dialysis is not going to be helpful in this setting in terms of long-term goals." He then offered that "Dr. Smith, myself, and Dr. Nadouri again discussed the fact that Mrs. Hamadani would greatly benefit from palliative measures at this point, and none of us would recommend proceeding with more aggressive measures including intubation and dialysis."

With all of that in his note, what stood out next was that he then reported that "the family does not, at this time, wish to have me write a DNAR order, that they prefer to wait until the decision to act must be made before giving permission not to proceed to intubation." Moreover, he reported a similar disposition regarding dialysis. And in the same breath (so to speak), he then wrote that he asked Dr. Nadouri to get a second renal consultant to take a look at Mrs. Hamadani in order to help determine if dialysis would be helpful.

After the usual listing of data, review of systems information, and so forth, Dr. Brouhkim's note ended with this:

"As mentioned above, we had a lengthy family meeting this morning. In addition to myself, Dr. Smith, ICU attending, Dr. Nadouri, nephrology consultant, nursing staff, and case management have all spoken with the family and discussed the fact that the patient's overall status is poor. Nonetheless, the family continues to request the patient be maintained as a full code and that dialysis be considered. We will continue to talk with the family and try to help them understand that these measures are not going to be helpful and most likely might be harmful, including shortening her life. The family fully understands these issues. All their questions have been answered. They remain at bedside and have told me that if the patient codes, at that point they will let the medical staff know if the patient should be intubated or not. Patient will remain at this point full code. I spent 8:00 am to 11:30 am this morning in the ICU providing care for Mrs. Hamadani."

"Yes," I thus replied, when Dr. Brouhkim asked me if I'd seen his notes form the past 2 days, "I have." "In fact," I continued, "I'm really intrigued by what you reported about your conversation from this morning, although that wasn't really the impetus for my call." I then told him about my encounter with Mr. Zaden and his sister several days prior and that I had "relieved" Steve of duty in this situation and thus would like to have a chance to sit with him and talk about what, if anything, I might be able to offer in terms of helping with this situation.

"That would be good," he replied, "although I'd like to wait and see what Rene Spector has to say." Dr. Spector, whom I knew was not only a nephrologist but possibly the most widely respected nephrologists in the hospital, must have been the "second nephrologist" Dr. Brouhkim had asked Dr. Nadouri to get. "He's usually good at seeing patients within a day, so maybe we could meet tomorrow. I'm planning on being over there again in the morning; will you be free then?"

I knew my schedule was open and so told him I would be. So we agreed to meet in the ICU tomorrow morning, and we would not only talk about what had gone on so far with Mrs. Hamadani's family, but what might be the next steps given whatever Dr. Spector might recommend. Thus our conversation came to an end.

Visiting with Mrs. Hamadani's Daughters

As I hung up the phone after my conversation with Dr. Brouhkim, I noticed that Nadira, the daughter I had met before, was walking over toward me. Having read about this morning's meeting, I wasn't sure what to expect as she approached. But as she neared, there was what I would describe as a "lightness" to her face, a change from the saddened countenance I had encountered when I met her initially. I stood up to greet her.

"Hello Dr. Finder, I am glad you have come by to see how our mother is doing. Please, come and meet my sister, Farzana." As I was now becoming accustomed with this situation, I was taken back somewhat by this. What, I wondered as we walked over toward Mrs. Hamadani's room, had motivated her to greet me as such and then ask me to meet her sister? As we approached the room, Farzana came out to greet us, and as she began to speak, I understood.

"Dr. Finder, it is a pleasure to meet you. My brother Samir has spoken of you and he is so grateful for your help in making sure that Dr. Moore no longer is a bother to us. Thank you so much."

She extended her hand as she spoke, which stood out as her sister, Nadira, had not. Indeed, Nadira was wearing a scarf and I was not sure if she was simply wearing a scarf or whether it was a Hijab. Farzana, on the other hand, could have walked out of one of those fashion magazines that populate physicians' waiting rooms and beauty salons given her skinny jeans, suede boots, flowery silk blouse, scarf around her neck, vest, and array of bangles on her wrists and earrings in both ears. She also seemed to be extremely observant, for in the second of hesitation I had in shaking her hand, she remarked, "I see you are a bit unsure whether it is acceptable to take my hand. For my sister, this is true, but for me, I do not live by those rules." As I grasped her hand in acknowledgement, I could not help but also note that her grip was firm.

I thanked both for their warm greeting, but then told them that, really, no thanks were due as I did not want to make their situation any more difficult than it was, for I had seen in Dr. Brouhkim's notes, and those from others, that the news about their mother was, I imagined, not what they wanted to hear.

"Is your mother still alive?", Farzana asked, looking intently and directly at me.

"Yes, she is, as is my father," I replied.

"Then you undoubtedly know," she continued, "how special it is to still have a mother with whom you can interact. As I know my brother told you, we have been blessed for the past 3 years to have been given a gift of these extra years to have our mother with us. None of us thought she would live this long, and Nadira and I have spent much of this time making sure that our mother is taken care of, that we do for her what she did for us, for all of us, even including our father, in the past. Although I have lived here in the United States for almost 30 years, I still hold fast to some of the values that come from our homeland. And respecting and caring for one's parents is high on the list. Unfortunately," and here she began to trail off, "many here do not share this belief."

Nadira, now standing next to her mother's bed, was holding her mother's hand in her's and gently stroking it. At the same time, she had her body slightly turned so that she was facing me and Farzana, and as Farzana was speaking, she nodded her head in agreement.

"Is it OK if I ask you some questions about your family?", I asked, wanting to be respectful of their space but also making the choice to take advantage of what seemed to be an openness toward me that I wasn't sure existed. But if it did, I did not want to miss the opportunity it provided to learn more from Farzana and Nadira.

"Of course, Dr. Finder," Farzana replied, again with the spark with which she had initially greeted me and then spoken.

Thus began what turned out to be a 45 min conversation with Nadira and Farzana. I learned that Farzana had initially come to the US in the mid-70s to go to college, and like many international students, decided to stay, attracted by the opportunities here. After the Shah fell in 1979, she had limited communication with her family until Samir had been granted permission to leave in the late 1980s, and then in the mid-90s, Nadira and their parents had come as well.

I also was told of their father's slow descent into dementia and how for the past few years, starting before their mother's cancer and continuing even until now, they had helped to take care of him. It was in this conversation that I thus learned that their father had been in a rehab facility for several weeks and was scheduled to come home any day now, and that they had not told him of their mother's hospitalization and so were worried what was going to happen when he was discharged and they brought him home but his wife was not there.

As an indirect learning, I saw that Farzana also seemed a bit dismissive of her younger sister, interrupting her on the few occasions when she tried to interject or add some detail to the tale Farzana was telling. Nadira, on the other hand, took this in stride. Both sisters, nonetheless, spoke only with a positive light about their brother, Samir, the youngest of the three. They expressed their concern, moreover, that unlike the sisters, both of whom, it turned out, were married and had children, Samir had yet to marry for he had not found a woman whom he believed his parents would accept. And since his mother's cancer was discovered, he had turned most of his energies, when not working as a salesman, toward making sure her care and her medical needs were met.

In short, I was presented a picture of a close-knit family in terms of there being a shared sense of commitment toward each other even as their lifestyles and ways of living differed (for instance, the religiosity of Nadira was more in line with what Farzana presented as her parent's beliefs, but she was nothing of the sort, and Samir was more like her than Nadira although he would occasional go to the mosque, especially during times when his mother was most ill).

The fact that I was willing to stand in the doorway of their mother's room, moreover, and listen to what they had to say did not go unnoticed. As our conversation wound down, both Farzana and Nadira remarked how grateful they were that I had shown an interest in their family and their experiences, and perhaps more importantly, that I had not told them how sick their mother was and how it was unlikely that additional intervention would make a difference to what, they didn't say explicitly but clearly hinted at in what they *did* say, was to come next, and soon at that.

We thus parted, and I left the Unit wondering whether we sometimes insist too strongly on having families speak directly about their loved one's deaths.

Meeting with Dr. Broukhim

The next morning, as we had agreed, I went to the ICU and met with Dr. Broukhim, and again contra to his reputation, he not only seemed to be pleased to have the chance to talk with me, but he was nothing short of explicit that he believed that the best thing for Mrs. Hamadani at this point was to shift to comfort only care.

"I think you know that I have a reputation for being very aggressive with my patients," he said several times, "and maybe it is more than others," he continued. "But when it comes to the point that I know I have pursued everything that might give them more life, I am also very blunt with them, and they know that if *I* say we are near the end, then it is true."

While these words could come across as arrogant and perhaps self-aggrandizing, they didn't. Rather, they were spoken each time during our conversation with a sense of care, that he would do whatever he could to help his patients as long as it would help them accomplish their goals and fit with their expectations. There was even a somewhat prominent degree of humility in his presentation that was not of the kind that one can fake or put on.

Perhaps more importantly, he was genuinely distressed over what was happening with both Mrs. Hamadani, as his patient, and with her children, as the ones he knew his patient cared about most, and thus for whom he too was deeply concerned. As I began to see, although it was not stated explicitly, part of what he was looking for in talking with me was reassurance that he was helping Mrs. Hamadani's children come to accept that he had few to no options left to provide for their mother.

More directly, he told me that late yesterday Dr. Spector had come by and decided that dialysis might be useful. While Dr. Broukhim did not think it necessary, he accepted Dr. Spector's assessment. In light of yesterday's conversation, this was not what I had expected.

Then the zinger: "Do you think this reasonable?" he asked.

'What a question,' I thought, given all that might be entailed in coming to any accurate sense of 'reasonable.' "Well, obviously, I must trust Dr. Spector here in terms of his judgment about the kidney and how dialysis fits into Mrs. Hamadani's current picture. I also know from what you've been saying in your notes and what the other consultants you've had weigh in, that in the big picture, dialysis won't change the ultimate outcome. Then there's the fact that this family seems to want to try whatever might hold out some sense of hopefulness for their mother to recover, even if only somewhat, and that's actually what she's been doing too for these past few years."

"I know there are a lot of folks," I continued, "who wouldn't hesitate a second and say that dialysis in this setting is completely uncalled for, that even offering it is problematic because, that it's a bad use of a limited resource and is a prime example of why our healthcare system is in the state it's in and why we need reform. For me, the details in the particular are the key, and it may well be that a few rounds of dialysis could help, give her a few more days to get over this hump. A lot turns on what the goal is."

"Do you know what Dr. Spector is after?" I asked. Broukhim replied that the thinking was that in the short-term, dialysis could help with the volume overload, hypernatremia and metabolic acidosis, and if the BUN could be brought down, there was a chance that her mental status might improve. "He thinks she may have some degree of uremic encephalopathy so this could help." He then turned to Spector's note from last night.

"He was pretty clear that, like you said, a lot turns on the goals; see." And with that he pointed to the end of Spector's note which read, in part,

"Renal replacement therapy is clearly indicated at the present time. However, this decision should be carefully considered with regards to both short-term and long-term expectations in medical outcomes. The patient may not tolerate due to hemodynamic instability. Unlikely to recover renal function, but will assist in dropping BUN, possibly improving mental status. I have discussed with patient's son and daughter, both eager to proceed if chance for improvement. I suggest they consider a short trial (i.e., 3 or 4 sessions) with the clear understanding that if her general condition fails to improve substantially, dialysis will be discontinued. They will discuss with other family before proceeding."

"I think with all that they've been through," Broukhim now said, "it's not unreasonable to see if we can wake her up and give them a chance to have a little bit a final time together. She's been a real fighter all along, and they've been so involved in her care, I think I owe them this."

For the fourth time in the 20 min we'd been talking, Broukhim's cell phone rang, he looked at the number, and then silenced the ringer. Then he said, "What I'd like to do is to give her a few more days and then have another family meeting with all three of the children and you. Of course, this is assuming that she remains stable between now and then. Does that sound OK with you?"

It was, and I said so. He then thanked me and as his cell phone began to ring again, this time he answered.

Another Few Days Interlude

Over the next few days, Mrs. Hamadani received several more sessions of dialysis and her mental status did improve somewhat, and there were points when she was purposeful. Removing the excess fluid also seemed to improve her respiratory function somewhat, although she continued to require Bipap most of the time; on occasions, her family took the mask off and her sats would slowly drift downward toward 90%, at which point they'd put it back on. The other main issue during this time was that her platelet count was dangerously low, down in the 10,000 range, and it was only with transfusion that they were able to see any improvement.

Several times during these days I stopped by and stuck my head in to say "Hello" to whomever was there, mostly Farzana and Nadira, although on two occasions Mr. Zadeh was also present. My aim in doing so was simply to keep tabs, much as Steve had done during prior hospitalizations. But unlike then, and unlike during the earlier part of this hospitalization, I did not inquire about whether they had thought more about CPR and DNAR or if there had been discussions of stopping the dialysis. Rather, I kept my focus on how they were holding up, especially the sisters who also had families for which they had responsibilities. I also asked about their father and the now unfolding plans as he was about to be discharged.

None of the conversations I had were as long as either of the priors ones, and for all of the initial warmth and openness that had been displayed when I first spoke with Farzana, these were much more truncated. I would not characterize the interactions as unfriendly or cold, nothing like that. They were always polite and gracious, but there was never a sense of their wanting to have any sort of sustain discussion. Their focus was clearly on their mother and anything that redirected their attention was of limited value.

During this time I also spoke with a variety of other care providers—nurses, respiratory therapists, the Unit social worker, and, of course, the physicians. With almost all of these conversations, there was little doubt about how these providers were experiencing Mrs. Hamadani's children. As Dr. Broukhim put it to me once when I saw him, the medical and nursing staffs were very "ticked off" by what he and Dr. Spector were "doing to" Mrs. Hamadani, and there was a resentment toward the family. Some of the staff were pointing fingers at other members of the staff, especially those who had developed a "give them what they want" approach toward the family whenever they requested extra attention. For instance, the fact that they were removing the Bipap mask themselves and questioning every intervention or interaction, be it drawing blood, changing tube feeds, or getting Xrays of her lungs. Dr. Spector's continued willingness to offer dialysis, of course, was the focus of most of the negative concerns surrounding Mrs. Hamadani's situation, and this was despite the fact that she was now slightly improved.

In talking with Dr. Broukhim, he was clear that he did not believe the improved mental status and stable hemodynamics that were attributed to the dialysis would last. Still, he was willing to defer to Dr. Spector. When I spoke with Spector, he reiterated what he'd written in his note: he'd reassess after 3–4 sessions of dialysis had been completed.

On the third dialysis day, I did have a somewhat longer conversation with Mr. Zadeh, which turned out to be significant for this reason: away from his sisters (I ran into him as he was leaving, and I was entering, the Unit, so we went and sat in one of the Meditation Rooms annexed to the family waiting area), he was quite explicit about his understanding of what was going on with his mother.

"You know, Dr. Finder, it has been a great blessing to have had these extra years with my mother, and I am deeply grateful to Dr. Broukhim for all that he has done. But I always knew that someday it would eventually come to end, that I will have to say goodbye to my mother. It is an awful feeling to know that, and even now, I still shutter at the thought of it." As he spoke this, he was slightly hunched forward, his hands crossed on his lap, his head slightly downcast. "I never think these thoughts when I am with my sisters for I must be strong with them. Our father, he has not been the strength in our family for some time, my mother was. And maybe she always has been, I do not know. But my sisters are devoted to her and have cared for her and have sacrificed for her." And then he just sort of stopped talking, and despite his large size and somewhat imposing figure, I was struck, really struck, by his vulnerability.

"Your parents would be very proud of you and your sisters for all that you have done, all that you continue to do, for them," I said, not sure if this was appropriate or if, rather, it was best to share the silence with him. I thus paused in the stillness of our sitting there, in the room.

And then it was gone.

"I have an appointment to which I must go," he said while starting to stand up. "Thank you for talking with me, Dr. Finder, I am grateful." We'd barely had a conversation but for a few words, really.

"I think Dr. Broukhim wants to get together with you and your sisters and me in a day or so; has he mentioned that to you?" I asked somewhat awkwardly since, if Broukhim hadn't, I may have erred.

"Yes, he has mentioned that. I will see you then."

And with that, Mr. Zadeh continued on his way. I went back into the Unit to see if there was anything new. In Broukhim's newest note I saw that he'd written that he and I were to meet with the family at 7:30 am the day after tomorrow.

The Family Meeting

I usually arrive in my office around 7:00 am, check email and get myself organized for the day. On this morning, I arrived even earlier so that I could get to the Unit a little bit before 7:30; it was 7:25 when I arrived there and Mr. Zadeh and his sisters were all in their mother's room. I sat down at the nursing station and waited for Dr. Broukhim. While waiting I pulled up Mrs. Hamdani's electronic record and read Dr. Teharani's, the consulting pulmonologist, note from yesterday. In it he mentioned that "upon examination of the patient, the patient is in agonal respirations," the result, it was determined, of the new Bipap masks not fitting well and hence not providing the necessary support; this was corrected and her status improved somewhat. He also stated that he discussed the possibility of intubation versus Bipap and that the daughter with whom he spoke—he did not indicate whether it was Farzana or Nadina—"implied that they are making decisions favoring not intubating the patient."

More interestingly, his noted continued, he had "extended my discussion to include intubation for respiratory failure even on Bipap which may be the case soon," and in this context, "the daughter was hesitant to make a decision and instead asked that serial blood gases be performed over night to assess the patient's condition" and that it would be "based on the results, the family would decide whether to intubate or not." He then noted that his interaction with the daughter "was pleasant and to the point" and that "her sister made a point to give a warm hello prior to leaving the room which was just prior to me entering."

And then the kicker:

"Due to my interaction with the patient's son the day before, especially his aggressive, abrasive and threatening tone and body language, complicated by his lack of faith in my recommendations, I gave the daughter a list of all active pulmonologists on the medical staff and offered to continue to treat the patient until they could find a replacement, at which time I will sign off. The daughter was grateful."

Obviously I'd missed something. But before I could pursue it further, Dr. Broukhim was standing next to me and he was making motions towards the family to come out of the room. I logged-off.

"Should we talk here?", Broukhim asked me as Mrs. Hamadani's three children approached the nurses station where I was now standing.

"No, it might be better to go and sit in one of the Meditation Rooms in the family waiting area," I suggested, and together, the five of us walked out of the Unit and headed to the Meditation Room in which I had previously briefly spoken with Mr. Zadeh.

We went into the room and sat down, the family sitting on one side, Dr. Broukhim and I on the other. Given the set up, I wasn't sure if I was there to help Dr. Broukhim or to facilitate a conversation, or both, or just to bear witness, so to speak. Accordingly, I waited to see what came next rather than assume that I was to begin this conversation.

It was, I discovered, the right choice, for Dr. Broukhim began without hesitation.

"You all three know that I adore your mother and I am honored to have been able to serve as her doctor these past few years. And I believe I have been able to help her, and I thank you for the opportunity to do so and to get to know you and your family in the process."

Already I could sense that this was a different kind of conversation than what I was used to, as Dr. Broukhim went on, using words such as "praise" and "respect" and "devotion" in reference to his interactions with Mrs. Hamadani and her three children who now sat across from us. And during this, they sat politely, one of them occasionally bowing their head slightly, all with hands gently folded on their laps. And when there was a pause, Mr. Zadeh began to thank Dr. Broukhim for all that he had done, and he expressed gratitude on behalf of his mother and his sisters. And as he spoke of his own appreciation for all that Dr. Broukhim had done, and the praise they all had for him, at times he held his hands to his heart and his eyes became slightly teary. At different points, both Farzana and Nadira shook their heads in agreement to what their brother was saying. For my part, I sat quietly and listened as, after this preface of what would be the conversation, Dr. Broukhim spoke once again.

He began to summarize all that had gone on with Mrs. Hamadani, beginning with his initial involvement as her oncologist. The prior 3 years worth of history were outlined fairly quickly, and so it was these past few weeks that became the real focus of his summary. Organ by organ, system by system, he presented all that was now failing: liver, lungs, kidneys, heart, brain.

"Her liver is now in the process of shutting down," he began, "and her lungs are unable to provide the necessary oxygen that keeps the body able to function. She's been on Bipap for over a week now, and typically, if a patient does not respond within that time-frame, we either elect to intubate or to withdraw care."

I cringed as he said "withdraw care" but now was not the time to suggest a different way of speaking.

"As you know, I had Dr. Spector review her renal situation which led to her having the several rounds of dialysis, and initially it seemed to make a difference. But after yesterday, he has decided that she is too sick for additional rounds, that whatever improvement it might potentially offer is far offset by the risks that her blood pressure would fall and we would not be able to maintain it."

"And in that regard, as for her heart, she is trying to compensate by working harder, but she can't keep up and we now have had to start her on medications to keep her blood pressure stable." This was a change from 2 days prior, but her children, having been in her room non-stop, already knew this, so it was only for me that this was news. "Although we're holding ground right now, if her blood pressure drops, we can increase these medications a little, but then there will be nothing more to do."

"And finally, with the shutting down of her liver and kidneys, her brain is now being crippled by the poisons these organs usually eliminate. When we take all of these together, and put it on top of her cancer, I am afraid that her time is very limited, possibly only days, weeks at best."

With these words, the picture he painted was dark indeed. But after having outlined all of this, he immediately shifted his focus, telling them that he simply wanted to ensure that they understood what was going on with their mother, not to change their mind about what to do, not to get them to say that they should withhold additional interventions or even withdraw any of the support currently being provided. "I know this is very difficult for you, and I want to make sure that you are fully in tune with what is happening so that you all can have the proper expectations for what is to come." With only a slight pause, he then stated that he was doing everything that he could to make sure that their mother was comfortable and not suffering, that above all else, "she has been such a lovely person and I do not want to do anything that will make her suffer."

This time there was a longer pause, and it was clear that now was the time for the family to ask whatever questions they had. Somewhat surprisingly, there were no questions. Rather, first Mr. Zadeh and then Farzana acknowledged their understanding of all that Dr. Broukhim had presented. Moreover, they thanked him for not only what he had done over the past few weeks, but for all of the care he had provided their mother during the years. Their tone was deeply respectful and there was not a hint of any sort of disagreement or discrepancy, difference or disconnect. As they spoke, I again harkened back to when Mr. Zadeh had asked me to stop Steve from seeing his mother: was this all as it seemed or was there manipulation occurring? After all, I still had Dr. Teharani's comments about how Mr. Zadeh had responded to him just 2 days ago and his own decision to remove himself from Mrs. Hamadani's case echoing in my thoughts.

And then, there it was:

"As you know, Dr. Broukhim, our mother has always been a fighter, a pillar of strength and determination and an inspiration for all of us, yes Farzana and Nadira, do you agree?" They nodded to their brother, and Nadira wiped her eyes. "And that is why, Dr. Broukhim, that our mother knew you were the right doctor for her because you too are a fighter. I remember the first day we came to your office and you told us about all the other patients in your waiting room, patients on whom others had given up but for whom you did not, and would not as long as there was hope." Mr. Zadeh's voice had that timbre I remembered as well, and with his size, the tone could easily come across as somewhat intimidating.

"That is why my sisters and I want you to continue everything that you are doing for our mother. And when the time comes that a decision needs to be made as to whether to do CPR or put her on a ventilator because she can no longer breathe, we will make our decision at that time, taking what the doctors and nurses tell us then."

Interrupting him, Dr. Broukhim acknowledged that Mrs. Hamadani was as Mr. Zadeh had stated and had strong views about fighting her cancer and that he wanted to be certain they understood that if they wished their mother to be coded then he would support them. But he did think it important for them to know that, "it is my professional recommendation that you not allow your mother to be intubated or cardioverted or to receive chest compressions as these interventions will not change the inevitability that awaits her, but they will likely cause her harm, which I do not want and I know you do not want."

Again, Mr. Zadeh spoke: "I think we all understand exactly what you are telling us, and I, and I believe my sisters too, appreciate the care and concern you show for our mother such that those are your recommendations. That is why, Dr. Broukhim, that we request from this point forward, we talk with no other doctors except you."

At this, Dr. Broukhim turned to me, literally, turned to face me, although he said nothing. It was as if he was now looking to me to help him, to decide whether this kind of arrangement was something to which he ought to agree. At least, that's how it struck me as he turned and looked at me as Mr. Zadeh concluded his comments.

Aware of the tension that had been developing between the family and other care providers, and given the fact that Dr. Broukhim had asked me to join him in this conversation and yet had not really invited me to participate in any substantive way until now, I wasn't quite sure what he now had in mind in turning to me. So I used this moment of redirection to restate all that I had heard over the course of their conversation, framing my remarks with the point that it was only by a kind of accident that I had become involved in Mrs. Hamadani's care, and as such, when it came down to it, I knew very little about all that was involved.

"But," I continued, "I do know this: you've got to trust one another since you're going to continue going through this together, one way or another. And I don't think I'm speaking out of turn in saying that there's been some, eh, lapse of trust with other physicians and care providers, so anything that can re-establish that trust is really important."

As I paused for just a second, I did a quick scan of the others to see if my use of trust as a theme was making any sense, and it seemed to be. And as I was about to continue, I suddenly found myself becoming once again aware of earlier conversations, only this time it was of what I had learned from Steve about his participation with Broukhim in that very first family meeting in which Steve had stepped into the breach when it looked as though all were on the same page, and what he said there had become the locus of their dissatisfaction with him. I decided I'd take the risk.

"When you have a really sick patient and a lot of different providers involved, there's always the difficulty of making sure that everyone is on the same page, so to speak, that what one person says is not misunderstood or confused by what others say or mean or intend. So I think if Dr. Broukhim is willing to play that role and have all the communication about what's going to be done for your mother flow through him, then that can work fine. But underlying this is the real issue, which is making sure that, as Dr. Broukhim has already said, you understand what's going on and that your expectations match, because the real problems are caused when we're not prepared for what's staring us in the face."

It all just came out and I wasn't sure if that was the right tact to take or not. But it became immediately clear that it was.

"You know, Dr. Finder," said Mr. Zadeh, "I think you are right. But the problem here is that everyone keeps telling me and my sisters all these bad things about what is going to happen to our mother as if we do not understand. But we do understand, we are not uneducated people. But is it too much to ask to please stop preaching about what is going to happen to our mother? We understand, we know, we get it!" His voice was now raised, and Farzana reached over as if to calm him, but he was in the grip of the moment, of release, perhaps.

"I do not want my mother to suffer, no one should ever want their mother to suffer. I do not need to hear 'we do not want your mother to suffer.' What I want is for my mother to be taken care of, and when the time comes to make a decision, my sisters and I will decide, and we will do what is best for our mother. This is not about me or you or Dr. Broukhim or anyone else. This is about my mother. Enough already, I understand all that you tell me, I understand all that Dr. Broukhim tells me, I just request otherwise. The doctors need to take care of my mother, the nurses need to do what they are supposed to do, and we, as the family, we will make the decisions that we need to make. OK?"

He paused and then added, "Please Dr. Finder, I do not wish to cause problems, and I apologize for raising my voice. But I do not ant to talk about this anymore and I do not want to talk with anyone else but Dr. Broukhim."

The End

How does one end a meeting such as this? There is no set way, nor, I believe, should there be. We often proceed as if endings need to be smooth and unitary, all the loose strings tied up together into an easily digestible resolution. But why should that be when the very context, and content, of such meetings concern a kind of coming apart, a dissolution, an undoing of a moment that has lasted possibly 83 years?

Mrs. Hamadani died just a few hours after this meeting. Her blood pressure bottomed out, and as Mr. Zadeh had requested, he and his sisters were asked, as their mother's heart rate went erratic and breathing became even more irregular, what they wanted to be done. And without hesitation, without dramatics, without conflict, they stated unanimously that they wanted to make sure their mother was not suffering, and they wanted to be alone with her and she passed from here to wherever she went, if any place at all.

PART TWO
CRITICAL RESPONSE TO THE ZADEH SCENARIO

Brief Summary of the Essays in Part Two

The titles of these essays in Part II already begin to demonstrate the range of significant issues raised in the Zadeh Scenario. In "Critical Self-Reflection as Moral Practice: A Collaborative Meditation on Peer Review in Ethics Consultation," Andrea Frolic and Sue Rubin generate an extensive set of questions for Finder. They probe the Scenario to suggest that ethicists "have an obligation to ask and debate the sometimes challenging questions raised by others' perceptions and expectations of us" (Frolic and Rubin 2018: 48). "For example," they ask, "is it our job to have the tough conversations with families, or to convince them to go along with the recommendations of the medical staff? Is it our job to contribute to reducing length of stay or to enhance patient satisfaction?" (Frolic and Rubin 2018: 48). They also argue for the need for clarity about the role for the ethics consultant, so that s/he doesn't get recruited to one side or the other in a perceived conflict, especially because the Zadeh Scenario "is a classic example of an ethical conflict. There are two parties who clearly disagree about what the right thing to do is regarding a patient's plan of care" (Frolic and Rubin 2018: 59).

In her essay, titled "Telling About Engagement Is Not Enough: Seeking the 'Ethics' of Ethics Consultations in Clinical Ethics Case Reports," Kelly Armstrong wants to know more about the patient, Mrs. Hamadani. Consistent with Frolic and Rubin's assessment, Armstrong's inquiry continues to show that the authorization for ethics consultation, the activities of the ethics consultant in the Zadeh Scenario, the significance gained in those activities, and the evident values expressed in such authorization and activities can all be traced along multiple networks of authority. Such authority may, at times, trail off to the unseen body of the long dying Mrs. Hamadani; at other times, those networks lead to Samir Zadeh and his grieving sisters; and at yet other times, the multiple networks of authority prominently lead to Dr. Broukhim and those other involved clinicians. Surveying that complexity, Armstrong suggests that the "fact that the children are always present and express feelings of love does not necessarily mean that they had a healthy relationship from the perspective of the patient, or that they are protecting and advocating for the patient's wishes rather than operating out of a different set of complex emotions or cultural understandings" (Armstrong 2018: 68). Nevertheless, although this family fulfilled their role for the decision-making process associated with their mother's care by understanding the information, integrating the family's and patient's values, and communicating their decisions regarding the clinical questions posed to them, additional issues remained. Armstrong introduces the frequently overlooked element of time, noting that "As a practical endeavor, facilitating accountable and ethically justifiable solutions means that as the clinical picture changes, so too may the ethically justifiable solutions" (Armstrong 2018: 71–2). Likewise, she says, "the unresolved issues in the narrative regarding the staff's distress and perception that the patient was suffering seem to be clear ethical concerns that warrant the reasoned deliberation of the ethics consultant" (Armstrong 2018: 71).

Anita Tarzian, in "Ethics Consultation for Mrs. Hamadani – A Focus on Process," shifts her focus to another set of assumptions incorporated in the idea that ethics consultation needs to be based in a standard set of procedures: "The point is that having a standard approach to ethics consultation does not mean that the ethics consultant must play the same role in each consultation – rather, the consultant should find out what the requestor wants help with and then clarify how the consultant proposes to help" (Tarzian 2018: 78). Like Armstrong, Tarzian also suggests that what is needed is a "strategy for determining how these decisions are made in a way that minimizes regrets for the survivors, meets fairness criteria, and addresses the moral residue and distress of the staff" (Tarzian 2018: 83). Tarzian provides considerable assistance to readers by introducing "the Persian concept of *T'aarof*, a ritual politeness code that governs behaviors between individuals of different hierarchies and imposes obligations to mitigate emotional distress by way of avoiding negative feelings" (Tarzian 2018: 78), an unspoken code that seems to be unstated and nonetheless quite evident in the interactions with Mrs. Hamidani's family.

In his contribution, "Ethics Consultation, Professional Praxis, and What It Means to Be a Consultant," James Hynds suggests that the basis of "ethics" in the situation that Finder has inherited from his colleague more closely resembles legal reasoning, in which the concerns of healthcare providers about standards of care and professional obligations are best understood through the dual lenses of medical standards and institutional policy and procedure. Although such an understanding suggests that the intention, let alone the effect, of ethics consultation should not be to persuade the family in this case, Hynds goes on to assert that the family needs to know from the attending physician just what the ethical reasons are – that is, based on professional values and standards – for not offering interventions and, more precisely, just when those values and standards will govern any actions taken, or not taken, and to explain to this family that there are procedures and policies to support those actions. Underscored by this clear argument made by Hynds are additional and directly associated ramifications regarding the role for ethicists, and he intends to use these as a basis to propose a more secure footing to support, even protect, their role. Hynds says, "if the hospital has a futility policy and Dr. Broukhim (or any other physician wants to invoke it), or Finder or Moore recommend that it be invoked, the reasons for the policy's existence, its substantive contents and the conditions for its invocation should have been carefully explained to Mrs. Hamadani's children as an instantiation and application of the institution's values and moral commitments, including a moral commitment to due process" (Hynds 2018: 96).

Perhaps Finder adopts a different kind of stance, while recognizing both a sort of institutional pressure and the concept of *T'aarof*. That possibility is acknowledged by Tarris Rosell and Brit Johnson in their chapter, "This May, or May Not, Be an Ethics Consultation". They suggest that "each of these initiators of ethics consultation was looking for help in stopping things they thought ought not to be done to their patient. Or they wanted help to stop family members who were trying to make clinicians do things they believed they ought not to be doing" (Rosell and Johnson 2018: 100). Then Rosell and Johnson ask a central question: "Is that what ethics consultants do? Stop things from happening?" In response they say, "Finder is giving care – and also showing compassion, patience, and tolerance, all of which are listed in the ASBH document as essential "traits" for health care ethics consultants (ASBH 2011: 32). He is kind and a good listener, in the normative manner of chaplains and counselors. He seems to care for and about this family. So this is morality, but is it ethics?" (Rosell and Johnson 2018: 102).

Reference

American Society for Bioethics and Humanities (2011) Core competencies for healthcare ethics consultation, 2nd edn. American Society for Bioethics and Humanities, Glenview

Critical Self-Reflection as Moral Practice: A Collaborative Meditation on Peer Review in Ethics Consultation

Andrea Frolic and Susan B. Rubin

Introduction

With "The Zadeh Scenario," Finder offers us a gift…a rich and thoughtful first-person account of the gradual unfolding of a specific ethics consultation conducted by a specific ethics consultant in a specific context. This is not your average case report, stripped to the bare facts and devoid of the ambiguity of real-time human interactions. It's also not simply an example of thick description, offering the reader a detailed account of the context out of which an abstract ethical dilemma has emerged, with the ethics consultant describing all from a distance, above the fray. What Finder offers and models for us instead is something entirely new and different. He offers us a case narrative into which he has chosen to place himself squarely and explicitly. And in the spirit of "peer review" he has generously revealed his own inner dialogue in response to twists and turns in the case, sharing his personal reflections as events unfolded, and his musings about various actions he took and choices he made in his role. By inviting us to ponder his story about the story of the case, he generously extends a gift to us: the opportunity to reflect on his—and therefore our own—consultation practice, and the opportunity to try a new kind of peer review.

One of the first things we were reminded of in reading Finder's narrative account of his practice is how, in any setting, individuals inevitably become "characters" based on how other people perceive them and the social roles that they play. This is no less true in ethics consultation, and proved to be an important entry point for us into the peer review process, particularly with respect to how the involved parties

A. Frolic (✉)
Office of Clinical & Organizational Ethics, Hamilton Health Sciences, McMaster University, Hamilton, ON, Canada
e-mail: frolic@HHSC.CA

S. B. Rubin
The Ethics Practice, Oakland, CA, USA

S. G. Finder, M. J. Bliton (eds.), *Peer Review, Peer Education, and Modeling in the Practice of Clinical Ethics Consultation: The Zadeh Project*,
https://doi.org/10.1007/978-3-319-90955-4_3

and Finder himself viewed his role and contribution. In "The Zadeh Scenario"—an account of a clinical case involving two ethics consultants, Finder and his colleague, Steve Moore—Dr. Broukhim plays the role of the "physician of last resort," a doctor beloved by his patients for enabling them to continue their fight against cancer when others insist on surrender. The family members who attend to the patient in this narrative through her long hospitalization (Mrs. Hamadani's son and two daughters) acquire the reputation of being not only lovely and devoted, but also difficult, intrusive, and bullying to staff. And as a visible part of organizational life, the ethics consultants too become "characters" in the social world of the hospital.

Through the narrative we see how both family members and clinicians assign motivations and attributes to ethics consultants that may have no grounding in (and, in fact, may be counter to) our own self-perceptions, roles and responsibilities, or lived practices. And this should be both a reminder and an invitation to us as individuals and as a field. As ethics consultants we tend to be more comfortable exploring other characters than turning the gaze back on ourselves. But critical self-reflection is necessary for both solid practice and meaningful peer review. In this chapter we argue that as ethics consultants, both individually and collectively, we must have a clear sense of our professional identity and a rationale for our practices (Rubin and Zoloth-Dorfman 1997). We have to take responsibility for independently establishing what our role is and is not, for defining what we will and will not do, and for setting and managing the expectations others have of us. Together as a field we have an obligation to ask and debate the sometimes challenging questions raised by others' perceptions and expectations of us. For example, is it our job to have the tough conversations with families, or to convince them to go along with the recommendations of the medical staff? Is it our job to contribute to reducing length of stay or to enhance patient satisfaction? Given the manifold pressures facing hospitals, it is not surprising that others will be happy to assign us roles that may align with the organizational priorities of the day. But it is incumbent upon us to be prepared to tell our own story, to articulate our own roles, to engage in continuous education about who we are and what we do, to correct potential misperceptions and to hold ourselves accountable. Sometimes we will disappoint or even anger others in the process. Nevertheless, we argue that we can and we must rise to the occasion.

But in our current situation, lacking the clearly recognizable trappings of a formal profession (like practice standards and credentialing processes) how do we even begin to articulate and defend our roles and responsibilities? How do we evaluate the quality and effectiveness of our unique roles as ethics consultants? How do we avoid simply being "good employees" or "trusted team members" by following the orders and priorities of our employers and clinical coworkers? How do we take independent moral responsibility for our practices when they are largely self-defined and self-monitored, and frequently invisible to even our closest colleagues?

Finder has afforded us the opportunity to experiment with peer review of a detailed case narrative as one method to enable rigorous reflection on these questions. By writing a detailed account of one of his ethics consultations—including his subjective experience of the consult, the clinical facts and social dynamics of the situation, and renderings of conversations over a period of days—we get a snapshot of his ethics consultation practice. The existence of this narrative is itself remarkable. As ethics consultants we spend a lot of time scrutinizing other health care providers' practices, but we don't turn that mirror on ourselves as often as we should. So much of our work is opaque to the public, to our employers, even to ourselves. When we tell people about what we do for a living we let the phrase "ethics consultation" roll off our tongues, but what does that really mean? What is the nitty-gritty, moment-to-moment manifestation of that work? The very existence of Finder's narrative points to a gap in our empirical knowledge of the field vis-à-vis what we are actually doing when we are doing ethics consultation (Frolic 2011). This narrative invites substantive and critical examination of "the ethics consultant at work in his native environment," affording the reader a rare glimpse into one person's lived practice.

This is a very different kind of peer review process from those involving evaluation of consult records or professional dossiers or even oral examinations using theoretical cases. It provides a clearer picture of actual practice (rather than merely demonstrating analytical prowess); however, it entails a great deal more exposure and vulnerability. We believe Finder's reflective piece offers an example of a practice that can and should shape the future of ethics consultation, especially now as we move towards professionalization and certification. We offer a deep bow of gratitude to Finder for his courage in making his practice…at least in this case…transparent to others. It affords us as a community of practitioners and scholars a rare opportunity to contemplate the challenges of mapping, molding and measuring the practice of ethics consultation. His moral commitment to transparency and self-examination is exemplary.

This chapter represents the composite reflections of both its authors. We use minimal references, drawing instead on our own practical wisdom acquired over the course of our careers, as peer reviewers tend to do. And we write in the first person plural rather than the third person; this retains the conversational and contemplative style of Finder's scenario, and compels us to own and personalize our observations about Finder's practice. In this way we share in the spirit of vulnerability he so eloquently and generously models in his narrative.

Our reflections are organized into two sections. First, we describe what we perceive to be the appropriate nature, role, scope and practice of an ethics consultant. Against this frame, second, we offer a close reading of "The Zadeh Scenario," focusing on Finder's portrayal of his role as an ethics consultant and the normative and procedural dimensions of his practice.

The Nature and Role of the Ethics Consultant: A Humble Declaration of Independence

If an ethics consultant were an animal…which animal would it be? The answer to this question—be it a platypus, a watch dog or a house cat—says something about how the respondent imagines the role of ethics consultation in contemporary healthcare. Similarly, the process of "peer review" is premised on the notion that ethics consultants not only have a clear role, but also *standards* against which a colleague's performance can and should be measured as good or bad. At this point in history, these standards are largely imagined, individual and idiosyncratic. Despite years of debate about this in the American Society of Bioethics and Humanities (ASBH) and by Canada's Practicing Healthcare Ethicists Exploring Professionalization (PHEEP), and despite the promulgation of documents like the Core Competencies (ASBH 2011) and the Model Role Description for Ethicists (Chidwick et al. 2010), in our view we still don't really have agreement on a number of basic issues that form the conceptual foundation of any real practice standard. Issues such as:

- What are we doing when we say we're doing ethics consultation? Facilitation? Decision Making? Mediation? Offering a kind, compassionate, supportive presence? Offering the perspective of the outsider—what Larry Churchill (Churchill 1978) named "the role of the stranger" years ago? Being an integral contributing member of the health care team, even "going native" in order to effect change?
- What goals do we have in mind? Ensuring the best care for the patient? Defusing conflict? Reducing length of stay? Reducing "non-beneficial treatment?" Drawing attention to the ethical dimensions of clinical decisions and helping to facilitate a thoughtful process of decision making grounded in careful and deliberate ethical analysis?
- How do we know if we are successful in meeting these goals? Should our evaluative measures focus on the experiences of stakeholders, including patient or staff satisfaction? Or should we favor more procedural measures, like whether the conflict was resolved or legal action was averted? Or should we concentrate more on longitudinal effects, like enhanced awareness of the moral dimensions of care and reduced moral distress?

In fact, without much empirical evidence to the contrary, we are guessing that the answers to these questions are likely to be widely divergent because we all enact our roles differently, with different goals in mind and with different degrees of success. That's precisely what makes any kind of standardization and meaningful peer review particularly challenging: by what standard are we measuring our peer's practices? Perhaps the first and most valuable step is to name our own biases about what we think are the hallmark features of ethics consultation, and to offer some account and defense of them. So we begin by articulating our answers to some of these questions, to declare where we stand, as a necessary preface to a critical peer commentary on Finder's narrative.

For us, the core commitments of the role of the ethics consultant that should guide his or her practice are:

1. **Role clarity**: The ethics consultant is not the *moralist* – and therefore shouldn't present herself as the knower or arbiter of all things good and right. Rather, it's the ethics consultant's job and unique contribution to support a deliberative process that includes: helping to identify the ethical dimensions of whatever

decisions or issues are giving rise to questions/concerns; identifying any underlying value conflict or value uncertainty; exploring and giving voice to the various perspectives of the different stakeholders/involved parties about the value conflict/uncertainty; facilitating meaningful discussion about the ethical questions at stake among them; and finally, offering guidance, recommendations or advice based on the information gathered and a consideration and analysis of the ethical appeals/issues at stake. It is crucial for us to be able to articulate how the role/scope of the ethics consultant overlaps with and is distinctive from other health professionals, including chaplaincy, social work, palliative care, risk management, etc. Ethics consultants must be prepared to articulate their distinctive role to stakeholders throughout the consultation process, and to defend the boundaries of this role when others attempt (intentionally or unintentionally) to shift or cross these boundaries (for example, by recruiting us as advocates for their perspective).

2. **Normative analysis**: While it's not the job of the ethics consultant to be prescriptive or determinative, in our view there is an inescapably *normative* dimension to the work. Our focus is on the "ought" questions. We're not there to simply name and comment on what is. Or to be passive observers. Or even to offer a supportive presence. We ought to have something unique and value added to contribute. And that contribution shouldn't be based simply on our ability to play well with others or make people feel safe, comfortable, and supported. It should be grounded in the discipline of ethics and should contribute something recognizably different and valuable to the equation. For example, while many health professionals might be able to describe a conflict about a treatment plan ("to resuscitate or not to resuscitate...that is the question"), the ethics consultant should be able to articulate the moral dimensions of the conflict and bring ethical theories (like consequentialism, deontology, or virtue ethics) and/or different methodologies (like principlism, casuistry, or narrative ethics) to bear on the situation. This is one of the unique contributions of ethics consultation to the social world of healthcare.

3. **Procedural clarity**: The ethics consultant ought to bring form, structure, and discipline to what otherwise might be an idiosyncratic and even freewheeling approach to the difficult questions that give rise to requests for ethics consultation. This form and structure not only ensures the integrity of the consultation process, but it also helps distinguish ethics consultations from all of the many other conversations and interventions that are likely taking place around a difficult case (such as patient/family care conferences or palliative care consults or conversations with the involved social workers or chaplains). By taking responsibility for keeping the focus of ethics consultation on the ethical issues at stake, and for bringing the tools, frameworks, and resources of the field of ethics to bear on the particular case, the ethics consultant helps ensure consistency and quality across ethics consultations. Though the methods of implementation employed to achieve those ends might vary, all ethics consultants ought to have ways to make their services known and clear mechanisms through which they can be accessed. And once accessed, we contend that ethics consultants must

take responsibility for defining the nature, structure, scope, and even pace of the ethics intervention. There should also be certain key recognizable components for which the ethics consultant should take responsibility such as: (1) Investigating and identifying what *is* the case? (What is the ethical dilemma? What is known factually? What values are at stake? Who is involved and what are their perspectives on the ethical dilemma?); (2) What *might* be the case? (What options have been or might be considered? What might be possible?); and (3) What *ought* be the case? (This involves exploring the normative dimensions of the case: What is the good/right/best thing to do in this case? Which possible next steps might be ethically defensible and which might not be? How do the options connect with the values of the various stakeholders? What is the consultant's recommendation?) Procedural transparency is an essential part of ethics consultation to engender trust and integrity. Thus, it is important for involved parties to understand that ethics consultations have beginnings and ends, and to know where they are in the process, and what the ethics consultant is doing and why along the way.

4. **Critical self-reflection**: Another hallmark of ethics consultation should be the creation of space for self-reflection about our own practices and about where we stand in the stories in which we get engaged. This is arguably an important practice for all health professionals. However, given that the "technical" dimensions of ethics consultation involve moral deliberation, conflict mediation and making space for epistemological pluralism, critical reflection on the question, "Where do I stand in this?" is particularly crucial: *What life experiences, commitments, allegiances, insider knowledge, and prior cases might be shaping my analysis of the case? How do my own histories and biases influence how I approach stakeholders, how I comport myself, what I say and when?* An ethics consultant, even one who is an outsider to the organization, cannot articulate the "view from nowhere" and all of us (being human) have particular moral blind spots. Humbly, we must acknowledge the influences on our behaviors and thoughts, and in some cases, we might even need to disclose these influences to others to ensure the integrity of the process.

Another form of self-reflection essential to ethics consultation involves the critical appraisal of our performance: *How well did I follow the procedures/norms that are supposed to govern my practice? How effective was I in staying true to my role and scope? What was the quality of my normative analysis?* Ideally, we should have access to multiple sources of data to appraise the quality of our work (client satisfaction surveys, anecdotal feedback, peer support, etc.), but we must also have the discipline to pause in the midst of our hectic days to contemplate: *"Was I true to my role...did I do my best...and did it make a difference?"*

The above summary of the hallmark features of the role of the ethics consultant represents a much-abbreviated version of the idiosyncratic standards that govern the authors' ethics consultation practices (though it must be acknowledged that we may each enact our roles in distinctive ways). Despite coming from different disciplines, practicing in different organizational contexts and in different countries, we readily agreed on these core features and used them to inform our analysis of Finder's narrative. We found ourselves remarkably in sync in terms of what surprised or gratified us in reading Finder's account of his role. What follows is a synthesis of our perspectives in the form of our peer review of Finder's case narrative, organized around the four core commitments articulated above.

A Peer Review in Four Parts

Role Clarity

There are numerous explicit and implicit references to the role and scope of practice of the ethics consultant in "The Zadeh Scenario." The consultant is asked to:

- follow the patient closely to try to provide support to the family
- provide more care for the family in these trying times
- delineate the ethical issues
- explain the clinical information
- get the family to make a decision or checking back with them re: their decision
- help the physicians have meetings with families
- defuse situations
- make suggestions (e.g. the ethics consultant was the one to recommend the n-g tube as a way to defuse one situation)
- translate between the physician and family
- make clinical referrals (e.g. the ethics consultant is the one who contacted the oncologist years prior)

And there are references to what the ethics consultant is *not* being asked to do, specifically to persuade or to be abrasive to the patient's family.

What was particularly striking to us about the narrative is how much Finder's involvement and role seems to be one of providing *emotional and personal support to the family*. We question whether that's the legitimate role of the ethics consultant. Yes, we should listen respectfully. Yes, we should acknowledge emotion. Yes, our presence is often supportive. However, if this is all we do, are we really doing what is more properly the work and legitimate role of other professionals such as chaplains and social workers, who are better equipped and trained to provide that specific kind of support? We think it's worth asking what happens to the distinctive contribution of ethics if the role is defined primarily as one of providing support.

It was interesting too that there's an explicit reference to the ethics consultant's role *not* being to persuade the family. Unfortunately, Moore (Finder's fellow ethics consultant) frequently found himself getting pulled into conversations between doctors and family members that seemed fundamentally about trying to persuade them. Given this context, and the fact that the family does not appear to have been explicitly told about the distinctive role of the ethics consultant, their perception that

Moore is there to advocate for the physician's perspective is understandable. And this is not an uncommon scenario. Ethics consultants are frequently enlisted when the team wants some added ammunition, if you will, and it is precisely at these moments that we think the ethics consultant needs to stand firm and in a place of integrity about what her legitimate roles and scope of practice are—to guard against being used to further others' agendas, however worthy or persuasive.

We think it is important to appreciate the fact that individuals in conflict naturally want to gather allies to their cause; without clear boundaries and the capacity to articulate them, it is easy for consultants to get "recruited" to one side or another. Or "scope creep" can occur, where difficult or unpleasant tasks are downloaded to the ethics consultant, such as the job of breaking bad news, or calming an angry family member, or saying "no" to someone who desperately wants a "yes."

This brings us back to the issue of expectations. The narrative excerpts the oncologist's note in which the desired contribution of the ethics consultant is described. In addition to hoping the ethics consultant will be able to provide support to the family, he also hopes the ethics consultant will be able to delineate the ethical issues involved in the care of this terminally ill patient. We agree that a focus on the ethical dimensions is intrinsic to the ethics consultant's role, but unfortunately we found that missing in the narrative. To put an even finer point on it, we want to argue that delineating ethical issues—while perhaps a necessary part of the ethics consultant's role/contribution—is also not sufficient on its own. The ethics consultant ought to be responsible for not only identifying but also actively engaging in discussion of the ethical issues, offering an analysis, and, where appropriate, making some recommendations.

Throughout the narrative we found instances of potential role confusion, either in terms of how the ethics consultants were conceiving their contribution or how others perceived them. This underscores for us the importance of being crystal clear about our unique role and contribution. We must be prepared to educate patients, families, and our colleagues about our role, and we must be constantly prepared to defend the boundaries of our role. In this way we can maintain a sense of integrity and protect against inappropriate uses of ethics consultation.

Not only can lack of clarity regarding the ethics consultant's role create confusion or unrealistic expectations, it can also create misunderstandings. For example, in Finder's narrative the family is described as feeling harassed by Moore's persistence in coming to check back with them. Clearly that wasn't his intention. But what in fact was he trying to do? What did he think he was doing anyways by "checking back" with them? And did he make that clear to the family? It seems like his intention was to see whether the family had had a chance to think more about the question he'd posed to them in a care conference, specifically, why was it that they were willing to proceed with aggressive interventions despite the various doctors' concerns? The question is a good one because it speaks to the family's motivation, goal, underlying intention, rationale and justification. These are all good to explore, but our suspicion is that it skewed the family's perception of Moore's role especially if it gave them the impression that they were to answer to him. This is a great example of how in the absence of early and explicit communication about the role and scope of the ethics consultant, confusion may ensue and various parties may actively try to recruit the ethics consultant to their "side" and then feel frustration when the ethics consultant doesn't perform according to their expectations. When the family first approached Finder, he could have taken that opportunity to tell them a little bit about the role of the ethics consultant in general; this may have helped to diffuse their frustration with his colleague Moore.

Although we may have a knack, as Finder clearly does in this narrative, for making connections or making people feel safe and comfortable and cared for, and although we may be recognized by our colleagues and patients/families for this capacity, it is important to ensure that our practices are reflective of and grounded in our actual role as *ethics* consultants.

Normative Analysis

An essential first step for an ethics consultant is to notice how those involved are describing the problems/challenges they are facing, and to invite and guide them to see their concerns through the broader lens of ethics. It's curious to us that in the narrative neither Moore nor Finder seems to take that next critical step. We are given a clear account of one physician's concerns but no separate account of the attendant ethical issues they raise. We quote the physician here:

> In addition to myself, Dr. Smith, ICU attending, Dr. Nadouri, nephrology consultant, nursing staff, and case management have all spoken with the family and discussed the fact that the patient's overall status is poor. Nonetheless, the family continues to request the patient be maintained as a full code and that dialysis be considered. We will continue to talk with the family and try to help them understand that these measures are not going to be helpful and most likely might be harmful, including shortening her life. The family fully understands these issues. All their questions have been answered. They remain at bedside and have told me that if the patient codes, at that point they will let the medical staff know if the patient should be intubated or not. Patient will remain at this point full code. I spent 8:00 am–11:30 am this morning in the ICU providing care for Mrs. Hamadani (Finder 2018: 31).

The team appears to believe that bludgeoning the family repeatedly with more clinical information and opinions will cause them to capitulate to their recommendations, something one would hope an ethics consultant would have noticed and drawn attention to. But despite 3.5 hours of conversation, and over 20 pages of narrative, many substantive questions remain unanswered that might have enhanced the quality of the moral deliberation around this case, and may have enabled the various "camps" in the case to gain insight into one another's perspectives and values:

- What is the family's goal for their mother's treatment? Can this goal be achieved? What is really driving their decision-making?
- What are the consequences to the patient/family/team of not having a clear plan for when her heart stops? How might this scenario play out?

- Who is the appropriate surrogate decision-maker? Who is the legal surrogate decision-maker?
- What are the obligations of the parties involved? Does local law articulate how families are supposed to make decisions for incapable patients? Are physicians obligated to get consent to withhold a treatment like CPR or can they write unilateral DNR orders?
- Does staff believe that the patient is being harmed by the family's decision-making? What is the nature of this harm?
- How do different health professionals perceive the case differently? How can they be supported to articulate and address their moral distress and to work together as a team?
- Mention is made of a hospital policy about medically inappropriate treatment. Why is this not applied in this case?
- And most importantly, where is the patient in all of this? What is her day-to-day experience like now? Who is she? What are her desires, goals and wishes? What did she say about her care when she was capable? How did she feel about the aggressive cancer treatment she received? Did she ever talk about dying? Did she recognize that her cancer was terminal? What gives her pleasure? What makes her life meaningful? How would she define quality of life?

When he sees the family again Finder states: "I did not inquire about whether they had thought more about CPR and DNAR or if there had been discussions of stopping the dialysis. Rather, I kept my focus on how they were holding up, especially the sisters who also had families for which they had responsibilities. I also asked about their father and the now unfolding plans as he was about to be discharged" (Finder 2018: 36). It is not clear why he steers away from engaging in analysis of the issues and focuses instead on emotional support. It is worrying that fear of upsetting the family or physician or anyone else would lead to the avoidance of precisely the questions and conversations that are most essential for the ethics consultant to engage, however painful, to ensure ethical patient care. The narrative does not offer any explanation for why Finder made the choices he did and what he thinks his role should have been in this case. It leaves us further wondering whether Finder would hold his behavior out as exemplary or, in retrospect, how he would adjust his practice.

Most disturbingly, the patient-as-person remains largely off-stage throughout the entirety of "The Zadeh Scenario," something one would expect the ethics consultant to be aware of and responsive to. Her inert body is a battle ground between the so-called loving family members (though we question whether it is really love or grief that is motivating their decisions) and the righteous, but impotent team that pushes decision-making onto the family and then resents them for the decisions they make. Her absence from the story provides a stark reminder of how quickly conflict can feed a downward cycle in relationships that can become self-reinforcing as patterns of communication are formed and what is most central to the conversation—the patient—is lost.

We believe that the essential roles of the ethics consultant are to identify the ethical dimensions of a case, to educate parties about relevant ethical standards, and to analyze the ethical dimensions of a case in light of the facts and relevant standards. In our minds, Finder seems to miss an opportunity to engage in the substantive work of ethics consultation. He offers support and empathy, but the crux of the conflict is neither named nor unpacked: that is, what treatment options are in the patient's best interests and in accord with her previously expressed wishes?

Let us clarify that we don't necessarily think that the outcome of this case is "wrong." We think Finder artfully portrays the merits of both sides of this conflict. We can't presume from this story that one side is correct and the other is incorrect, and this quality of the narrative alone is admirable. For in the genre of case reports, ethics consultants frequently vilify one side and valorize the other. However, we remain frustrated that we don't have sufficient information to judge the ethicality of the outcome of the case, because key questions seem never to have been addressed. It is this lost opportunity to engage in substantive analysis that is the source of our greatest frustration and concern in reviewing "The Zadeh Scenario."

Procedural Clarity

Having procedural clarity about the various phases of ethics consultation can help ensure appropriate attention to the normative dimensions of the consultative process, keep the ethics consultant on track and set clear expectations for interactions between the consultant and the various stakeholders. The lack of this kind of procedural clarity was notable in Finder's narrative. At the same time, Finder and Moore seem to share certain process elements in their approach to ethics consults including:

- Talking to stakeholders one-on-one
- Attending family meetings, primarily to listen and ask questions and offer suggestions
- Reading the patient's medical record
- Documenting in the patient record

And there seem to be some admirable features of Finder's practice including the following:

Mindful, Non-Judgmental Respectful Listening A commitment to this quality of listening seems to be an integral part of Finder's practice. The narrative is full or references to Finder listening and listening well. We agree that making it a practice to listen deliberately and thoughtfully is certainly an important building block in establishing trust and rapport which may be necessary in order to successfully delve into the harder material. However, we would argue that listening is a necessary but ultimately insufficient skill/contribution of the ethics consultant. Finder's narrative left us concerned that he might have risked creating the misimpression that the ethics consultant's role is simply to listen as opposed to being an actively engaged participant contributing something unique to the process/case. That being said, we are painfully aware of how easy it is to make a misstep by prematurely jumping in with pronouncements/opinions based on incomplete information in the interest of demonstrating one's value in a difficult situation. It's also possible to make the mistake of accepting the mantel of the "moralist" who has some direct access to the truth and whose job it is to enlighten everyone else. And so we commend Finder for making neither of these mistakes.

Continuity of Care Another feature of Finder's practice seems to be "following cases." This is something that was striking for us and raises real questions about the role and scope of practice as well as the kinds of expectations such a practice may foster. Finder makes reference to relying on the electronic medical record to notify him when patients the ethics service has been involved with in the past are readmitted, presumably so ethics can "check in" with them and continue to "follow" the case. While this may provide some benefit in cases involving recurrent ethical conflicts, this is also a marker of how much Finder's ethics practice is embedded/nested in a medical model. We worry this could lead to some inadvertent role confusion (What exactly is the ethics consultant contributing by "checking in" on a previous case?), as well as potential violation of the patient's privacy.

Visible Integration "The Zadeh Scenario" exemplifies the visible integration of the ethics consultant into the clinical context of patient care. Finder is obviously not spending all of his time in an office far removed from patients, which we both applaud. He doesn't expect people to come to him, he goes to them. This allows him to see and understand the context of care, to observe interactions between parties in a "natural" environment, and to be more meaningfully accessible. This is particularly evident in Finder's attention to geographical space and the context of conversations. Such integration into the flow of clinical care can enable: relationships of trust with clinicians; personification of issues that otherwise can be very abstract; better fact gathering and direct communication with stakeholders. But it also potentially raises the host of concerns addressed in the literature about "going native," including losing critical distance/perspective and cementing alliances that might disadvantage certain stakeholders in a case.

But as noteworthy and positive as each of these elements of Finder's described practices are, we think there are downsides to them as well. What strikes us most about the methods described are their *informality* and their seeming disconnection from what we see as the essential and unique contribution of the ethics consultant –the focus on the normative questions raised by the case. The ethics consultant is portrayed as one who wanders in and out of units and meetings, whose primary role apparently is to "check on things" and to "see what is happening" and "offer support." But what does all of this checking and seeing really contribute? Finder himself expresses concern over the lack of clarity in his role during his last family meeting: "Given the set up, I wasn't sure if I was there to help Dr. Broukhim or to facilitate a conversation, or both, or just to bear witness, so to speak. Accordingly, I waited to see what came next rather than assume that I was to begin this conversation" (Finder 2018: 38). We believe this case demonstrates that without a clear consultation process—a discrete beginning, middle and end, and clear markers along the way—the work of normative analysis and moral deliberation and the intended role of the consultant can easily get lost in the drama of the conflict.

This case is a classic example of an ethical conflict. There are two parties who clearly disagree about what the right thing to do is regarding a patient's plan of care. Not all consultations present this way, but such cases seem well-suited to bioethics mediation or a formal committee consultation process. A formal process serves several purposes:

- It allows multiple parties to hear one another simultaneously and to communicate directly with each other. If the ethics consultant only talks to one party at a time, they are in danger of triangulating relationships and compounding the miscommunication that so often happens in fragmented hospital care.
- It allows for asking difficult questions and telling difficult truths to one another in a supportive setting.
- It can ensure that all parties' values and concerns are heard, through facilitation by a neutral person.
- It can focus primarily on a narrow function/goal, that is, naming and examining the ethical dimensions of the case, as opposed to building relationships or information-sharing—the typical functions of family meetings.

These functions cannot be fulfilled without some formalization of both the ethics consultant's role and process. In a few places it is mentioned that the nurses are deeply distressed about the "futile" care being provided to the patient. What is the role of the ethics consultant in addressing this distress? It is impossible to tell from this narrative if and how the voices of the bedside staff were included in the consultation process. For example, in a formal consultation process, the ethics consultant could invite a member of the nursing staff to share her perspectives on the patient's experience of her life, its quality, its challenges, etc. along with the concerns of the bedside caregivers. In addition, the ethics consultant could provide a case debriefing or similar process for nursing staff to articulate their values and concerns (either concurrently or retrospectively) to address their moral distress and to enhance their understanding of the ethical dimensions of the case. This could be a unique contribution of the ethics consultant to alleviate the mounting tensions in the ICU, to build capacity and to address the potential fall-out of this case after the patient has died.

But this narrative points to a second procedural challenge. It does not appear that ethics consultation in this case contributed to any positive outcome, beyond a good relationship between Finder and the family. It did not enhance relationships between stakeholders or support a deeper understanding of their diverse moral perspectives (if anything it appears that the nursing staff was increasingly alienated throughout the process). It did not result in a clearer plan of care for the patient. It did not result in the patient's voice being heard and honored. From an administrative perspective, was the benefit gained worth the cost? It is difficult to imagine how Finder and

Moore would measure the quality of their consultation process, apart from whether people liked them or valued their support. But what about other quality markers like ethicality, adherence to process measures, or capacity-building? In fact, without a clear beginning, middle and end to the case, it is impossible to define any outcomes at all or to make judgments about the effectiveness or quality of the consultation as a distinctive contributor to a particular case.

Critical Self-Reflection

"The Zadeh Scenario" has given us an opportunity to reflect on and deepen our understanding of the necessary components of a rigorous and meaningful process of self-reflection. If we are to hold ourselves accountable to continually reflect on and improve our practices, we need to apply rigorous normative analysis to ourselves and to our practice, just as we do for our consultation cases. In other words, it is not enough to be able to describe to ourselves or even to our peers what we did or what we do. Just as we offer a response to the classic question of ethics when we are called to offer ethics consultation in specific cases – what is the right/good act and what makes it so? – so too ought we be able to offer a normative defense of our practice – what was the right/good way to approach this case, what makes that so, and how well did we do in upholding that standard? We need to be able to offer an account and a defense to ourselves and to our peers, not only of what we did, but *why* we did it and why we thought it was the good or right thing. We need to be able to describe: our thinking and underlying rationale; the beliefs, assumptions, and biases that guided our choices; the tradeoffs or compromises we may have consciously or unconsciously been willing to make; and how we might have allowed ourselves to be impacted by the external constraints under which we have been asked to practice. Finally we need to be able to critically appraise how well we managed the core commitments that we argue should guide the practice of ethics consultation: role clarity, normative analysis, procedural clarity and critical self-reflection.

In reviewing Finder's narrative, we are struck by how he seems to have shied away from that sort of critical normative analysis both about the case itself, and about his own practice. Though he is clearly committed to self-reflection in that he has offered a rare and welcome look into his internal thought processes, and has unabashedly and without reservation invited public peer review of his practice, for some reason he stops short of sharing his own self-appraisal of his practice. He offers description without analysis, and as reviewers, it has left us wanting more. We don't have any sense of whether Finder would endorse or criticize his conduct in the case. We don't get an account or defense of the role he chose to assume, decisions he made about engaging or not engaging the normative questions raised by the case, or procedural choices he made in organizing his involvement in the case. And it makes us wonder why. Is Finder withholding his own commentary so as not to bias or influence the conversation or process of peer review? Is he hesitant to presume consensus about the standards to which we should hold ourselves accountable and is therefore at a loss for how to responsibly critique his practice? Do a different set of questions altogether arise for him in evaluating his practice, making the questions we've raised less compelling or relevant for him?

Whatever the reason, the absence of normative self-reflection in the narrative Finder has offered highlights the necessity of incorporating it as a key component of a process of meaningful self-reflection. And to create accountability, that process of reflection can't exist in an insular, self-referential vacuum. That is where we must support one another as colleagues in the field, to create and hold the space for that sort of reflection, to demand it of one another, and to create safe opportunities for peer review so that we can hold our practices up for others to examine and evaluate, as Finder has modeled.

References

American Society for Bioethics and Humanities (2011) Core competencies for healthcare ethics consultation, 2nd edn. American Society for Bioethics and Humanities, Glenview

Chidwick P, Bell J, Connolly E, Coughlin MD, Frolic AN, Hardingham L, Zlotnik Shaul R (2010) Exploring a model role description for ethicists. HEC Forum 22:31–40

Churchill LR (1978) The ethicist in professional education. Hast Cent Rep 8(6):13–15

Finder SG (2018) The Zadeh Scenario. In: Finder SG, Bliton MJ (eds) Peer review, peer education, and modeling in the practice of clinical ethics consultation: the Zadeh project. Springer, Cham, pp 21–42

Frolic AN (2011) Who are we when we are doing what we are doing?: the case for mindful embodiment in ethics case consultation. Bioethics 25(7):370–382

Rubin S, Zoloth-Dorfman L (1997) Navigators and captains: expertise in clinical ethics consultation. Theor Med 18:421–432

Telling About Engagement Is Not Enough: Seeking the "Ethics" of Ethics Consultation in Clinical Ethics Case Reports

Kelly Armstrong

Introduction

"The Zadeh Scenario," a wondrously rich narrative generously shared by Finder, walks the reader through the interactions of an ethics consultant during a case. In this telling, Finder appears deeply cognizant of how memories can be affected by subsequent decisions and experiences. Hence, it is important to note that many key parts of the narrative – if not all of it – were captured concurrently or in close proximity to the actual events, thereby revealing the factual and normative obscurity that unfolds over the course of an ethics consultation. Finder's polished skills of careful attention and mindful appreciation in recounting the "doing" of an ethics consult thus provide something of an anthropological account – telling us who went where and the content of several weighty conversations – rather than what might traditionally be expected from an ethical analysis of a case presentation.

Importantly, though, this accounting exposes the difficulty of abstracting moral understanding from a description of the actions of the involved parties. At the same time, the narrative also reveals an important limitation of case presentations, namely that they are generally presented as a concrete case in time with a firm beginning and end. For all its richness, much of the information that is needed to assess what is ethically important or problematic in the consult falls outside of the scope of the narrative we have before us. This deficiency may partly lie in the fact that like many ethics consults, the ethics consult in which Finder finds himself has an unclear beginning – did it begin 3 years ago when an ethics consult was called by the neurologist; did it begin during subsequent hospitalizations when Dr. Moore was approached by concerned individuals involved in Mrs. Hamadani's care; did it begin

K. Armstrong (✉)
Center for Clinical and Organizational Ethics, Virginia Commonwealth University School of Medicine Inova Campus, Falls Church, VA, USA
e-mail: kelly.armstrong@inova.org

S. G. Finder, M. J. Bliton (eds.), *Peer Review, Peer Education, and Modeling in the Practice of Clinical Ethics Consultation: The Zadeh Project*,
https://doi.org/10.1007/978-3-319-90955-4_4

during this hospitalization when Dr. Broukhim requests the consult from Dr. Finder's ethics colleague, Dr. Moore; or did it begin when Mr. Zadeh approached Dr. Finder outside the hospital? Moreover, is Finder picking up where Dr. Moore left off, or is he in some way beginning the consultation anew alongside the new relationship he seeks to establish with Mrs. Hamadani's family? The narrative of "The Zadeh Scenario" is not clear on this point, but it is an important issue to consider as we consider the activities of the ethics consultation we have before us.

Preparatory Elements of a Consult

After Mr. Zadeh approaches Dr. Finder outside of the hospital passionately explaining that his family no longer wants to interact with Dr. Moore or even have Dr. Moore check in on the patient, one could have expected the narrative to turn to a discussion of the difficult ethical implications of carrying out an institutional ethics consultation without the involvement of the patient or her family. Finder acknowledges that he didn't think it was "appropriate to force family members to talk with ethics consultants even if we continue to meet with members of the patient care team" (Finder 2018: 26). Yet, he begins preparing for what "was looking to be a very interesting consultation" (Finder 2018: 29), assigning the role of ethics support for staff and other care providers to Dr. Moore while preparing to take over the consultation with Dr. Broukhim and the family himself. Unfortunately, the rationale for this move is never fully explained in the narrative. Was the family saying they did not consent to the ethics consultation process, or merely saying that they no longer wanted to speak with Dr. Moore? This is an important distinction with wider implications regarding the goals of ethics consultation, issues of consent, and the dual role of ethics consultation in the care of patients and in supporting the processes of the institution.

As Finder prepares to take over the consultation, the narrative illustrates many important elements of preparation that are critical to a successful consultation process. Before any analysis or clarification can begin, the specific details of the case frame the issues and diligent research of the medical record along with conversations with care providers provide a necessary understanding of the clinical, contextual and social factors that ground important values expressed by the patient, family and caregivers. Thus, it is important that we see Finder begin his participation in the consultation process by pulling up the patient's electronic medical records to better understand what had been happening not only medically, but also in regard to the social dynamics surrounding Mrs. Hamadani's care. Only after this grounding does he call the original consultant on the case, Dr. Moore, to discuss Dr. Moore's understanding of what had happened during this and previous hospitalizations. The conversation touched upon not only Mrs. Hamadani's medical situation, but also important information from Dr. Moore's conversations and interactions with her family, her physicians, and the nursing staff. Significantly, we also see Dr. Moore's analysis of those interactions in regards to their emotional content and the perceived motivations of the persons involved in those specific interactions.

Before going to the Unit, and thus making his presence known as a person now involved in the patient's case, Finder notifies the attending physician, Dr. Broukhim, that both he and Dr. Moore were now involved in Mrs. Hamadani's case. This is appropriate for a number of reasons. The initial request for ethics assistance did not come from the patient or family, where it may be appropriate to first speak with the requestor of ethics assistance to determine the nature of the ethical question or issue. Rather, it was Dr. Broukhim who had requested Dr. Moore's assistance. Since the process of ethics consultation is an ongoing process of dialogue and deliberation, as a matter of respect for the relationship between patient and physician as well as a matter of practicality, attempts to inform the attending physician should occur near the beginning of the consultation process, and whenever possible, before any conversation with the patient or family. The attending physician is the person ultimately responsible for the care of the patient and as such, he or she should be aware of matters that may affect the patient's care and disclosure of the patient's confidential information. Furthermore, the physician may have key information regarding any questions or issues that may have presented themselves. Notification is not the same as asking permission. In order to empower the moral agency of all persons involved in the ethical provision of care, individuals should feel that they can request a consult when they feel it is appropriate, without fearing retribution or having their concerns vetoed by the physician.

Although the narrative initially noted that Finder planned to discuss the case with the ICU staff as well as Dr. Broukhim, we are only told about the discussion with Dr. Broukhim. It is unclear if Finder intended to meet with the patient or clarify his role with the family. As a matter of general practice, one should always try to meet with the patient whenever possible. Ethics consultation is undertaken on behalf of a real person, not an abstract construct gleaned from written or oral accounts. Therefore, rather than relying on second or third-hand descriptions of the patient, it is a commendable aspect of practice to meet with the patient regardless of their decisional capacity or physical state in order to have an independent picture of their mental and physical circumstances. This is not only a matter of respect, it often yields surprising and useful information missing from the accounts of other persons.

In regard to clarifying Finder's role with Mrs. Hamadani and her family, opinion 9.115 of the AMA Code of Medical Ethics states that "in general, patient and staff informed consent may be presumed for ethics consultation" (AMA 2014). However, Mr. Zadeh, Mrs. Hamadani's son, had made clear his desire to not speak to the ethics consultant, Dr. Moore, or have him interact with the family any longer. There is no reason to presume that he intended, or would even agree to have, Finder replace Dr. Moore as the ethics consultant in his mother's case. When Mrs. Hamadani's daughter Nadira approaches Finder on the unit and invites him to meet her sister Farzana, the encounter appears primarily social, motivated by their gratitude for "making sure that Dr. Moore no longer is a bother to us" (Finder 2018: 32). Although Finder had begun his role as an ethics consultant on the case, he does not make this clear to the patient's daughters during their exchange in the patient's room. Under the guise of a social exchange, Finder asks them questions about their family, "making the choice to take advantage of what seemed to be an openness toward me that I wasn't sure existed, but if it did, I did not want to miss the opportunity it provided to learn more from Farzana and Nadira" (Finder 2018: 33). Ethics consultants can learn a great deal about the history and social dynamics of a family through casual conversation and observation, and in some situations this may be preferred over a formal interview-style of dialogue. Yet, the issue of informed consent looms large in this situation. Even though the patient's daughters freely exchange information with Finder regarding their family and their lives, one has to wonder if they would have been so forthcoming if they understood him to be gathering information based on his role as Dr. Moore's replacement.

As Finder "takes over" involvement with the family, his visits with the family exhibit features more in line with those of a supportive presence or respectful listener, rather than a facilitator or mediator of value conflicts or uncertainty. Yet, if a responsibility in clinical ethics consultation is to remain acutely aware of the multiplicity of power differentials inherent in social and clinical interactions, and to attempt to limit vulnerability or coercion in those interactions, then the mindful, nonjudgmental listening that formed the core of Dr. Finder's interactions with the family could be understood as a responsible starting point for any potential future moral engagement. This is especially true given the psychosocial dynamics associated with the patient's care. Despite clear and unvarying instructions regarding their wishes for CPR, the family repeatedly reacts to the perception that they were being pressured to make a different decision. Mr. Zadeh says "he did not visit, he simply came to get us to say what he wanted to hear," and at one point highlights feelings of discrimination, asking "Did Frank Sinatra's family have to have these conversations?" (Finder 2018: 26). Not all consultations require this type of supportive interaction to foster trust, however in this case respect for, or even tolerance of, the role of the ethicist to facilitate meaningful discussion regarding the ethical dimensions of the case had severely diminished.

Despite the appearance of the family's deeply held convictions, the patient's complex medical needs may at any time have led the family to have doubts or questions about their commitment to their stated goals and plans for the patient. Finder's continued supportive presence provided the family with a safe and meaningful forum to reflect upon any issues or concerns they may have had, in their own time, without exacerbating potential vulnerabilities they may have felt. With a strong possibility that the patient's clinical condition would warrant another contingent of decisions subjected to substantive critical examination, Finder's attempt to establish a relationship with the family addresses the fact that he was coming to the encounter as a stranger – a stranger who nonetheless had the power to engage in focused and critical questioning of the family's deeply held moral commitments. From the family's perspective, deeply delving into and analyzing their decisions may have seemed to yield only the potential for further psychosocial disruption with little concurrent upside. It is therefore appropriate, and perhaps desirable, to give the family the space and time to understand and adjust to both the current clinical picture and Finder. While it may leave the reader of the narrative yearning for Finder's more active engagement of the myriad ethical issues of the case, one could argue this supportive interaction with the family was a necessary foundation to what was, at the time, an unknown constellation of future events.

Despite these initial investigations and conversations, it is both surprising and worth noting that Finder fails to explicitly engage in other preparatory elements that one would expect to find, such as an exploration of what is known regarding the patient's wishes, her legal decision-maker, or any details that have come to light regarding the lived experience of her illness and family life.

The Missing Patient

The patient's autonomous right to participate in conversations about her care, and to make informed decisions about that care, has a long-standing history in American jurisprudence and medical ethics. It is therefore common for case reports in clinical ethics to begin and end with a focus on the patient and the patient's wishes and goals. When the patient lacks decisional capacity, the patient's wishes must be gleaned from past statements and/or expressed by a legally authorized proxy decision-maker. Mrs. Hamadani may be well-represented through the wishes and support of her family, yet the extent to which her family represents the patient's wishes remains unclear, as does the question if they represent her legal decision-makers under state law. Many states limit the types of decisions that can be made by a patient's legal representative, or have restrictions based on what type of decision-maker is providing the consent (such as power of attorney for healthcare, guardian, or a non-patient-designated individual). It is therefore important to better under stand the broader ethical, legal and social context of the role of these decision-makers and any limitations that may exist regarding decision-making.

Despite a narrative that in some respects covers 3 years of time, in "The Zadeh Scenario," Mrs. Hamadani never makes a first-person appearance. The silence of the patient's voice is distressing, not only because the right to consent to or refuse treatment lies with the patient (even when that right is executed on her behalf by a proxy decision-maker), but also because we have a sense that she may have been decisionally capable during significant portions of her treatment and thus able to participate in shared decision-making regarding her treatment and goals. She was, after all, still at home taking care of her husband (he had been diagnosed with dementia) – presumably not the act of a woman unable to make decisions. Over the course of her multiple hospitalizations did the physician, the ethics service, the palliative care service, or anyone else make an attempt to engage Mrs. Hamadani in advance care planning for her terminal illness? An explicit inquiry into and analysis of her values, her decisional capacity, her expressed or previously expressed wishes, her personal goals, or even the identity of the person she would choose as a proxy decision-maker are lacking. Instead, there is only a reflected appearance viewed through the lens of her medical condition, reports of interactions with her family by the physicians and consultants, and a few reports of her history (not her wishes) provided by family members. Of course, some patients do not discuss their illnesses or express their wishes. It is especially at these times that the ethics consultant can be helpful to clinicians and family members in guided discussions to uncover and explore the patient's wishes based on past statements or personal preferences and disposition.

It is concerning that "The Zadeh Scenario" narrative fails to explicitly identify and analyze whose wishes are being expressed, instead focusing on the role of the patient's children in decision-making. For example, the case begins with the account that the patient's son, "Mr. Zadeh, and his sisters... found an oncologist who was willing to pursue aggressive treatments" (Finder 2018: 22) after his mother had been diagnosed 3 years ago. There is no mention if the patient had chosen to fight the illness with the support of her children, or perhaps that she had chosen to defer to her children's desire to get a second opinion. Going further, the original ethics consultation called by the neurologist cites the neurologist's belief that "the *family's* request for aggressive intervention" was inappropriate, and that the patient's *son and daughters* had shouted the physician out of the room and fired him (Finder 2018: 22, emphasis added). The rest of the Scenario reveals that physicians wanted assistance speaking with the *family*, that treatment decision meetings were held with the *son and daughters*, and the *family* was asked to make decisions regarding their mother's care (emphasis added). When Finder becomes involved, he appears to continue this trend. There is no mention of the patient's decisional capacity as he begins checking her chart and speaking with staff about the patient's medical condition. When he moves on to discuss with Dr. Moore the conversations Dr. Moore had with the patient's physicians, he does not ask about any interactions with the patient but wants to know "more about [Dr. Moore's] interactions with Mrs. Hamadani's children" (Finder 2018: 28).

Thus it is important that we do not know the patient's perception of her relationship with her children. The fact that the children are always present and express feelings of love does not necessarily mean that they had a healthy relationship from the perspective of the patient, or that they are protecting and advocating for the patient's wishes rather than operating out of a different set of complex emotions or cultural understandings. Certainly, it would have been ethically permissible for Mrs. Hamadani to request that decisions be made by her children, or even to request not to be a part of discussions about her care and treatment. However, by failing to mention any conversation with the patient during which the patient made such wishes for non-participation known, it is troubling that the case appears to presume that she did not wish to be involved in decision-making, or that her wishes were adequately represented by her children. What we are told is that the family is Persian, and there is a suggestion that cultural elements may "have been part of what was at play" (Finder 2018: 29). However, a commendable sensitivity to the patient's and family's cultural traditions would not justify a presumption that the patient wished to defer decision-making to her children or that she wished to entirely forgo any participation in discussions. As a result, the information we are given to reflect upon regarding what may constitute morally appropriate treatments or outcomes is questionable since it is the direct result of a different set of questions – what the care team feels is in her best interest, and the questions asked of the patient's family regarding their wishes regarding treatment decisions.

The distress of the patient's silence is compounded by the relative silence and stereotypical treatment of the patient's daughters. It is only the patient's son who is given a last name, is consistently referred to by his formal name "Mr. Zadeh," and who voices instructions to the care team in the narrative. While he appears to be well-supported by his sisters and there is no obvious discord between the family members, none of the female characters' opinions regarding treatment independent of Mr. Zadeh's interpretation are explored. Thus we cannot know if there was consensus among the patient's children regarding treatment or if they were unified in their understanding of their mother's wishes. Instead, the narrative never asks the question of whether Mr. Zadeh speaks for the family, and both the patient and her daughters form a silent chorus for Mr. Zadeh. In the absence of any discussion of the patient's views, her daughters' views, or of who is fulfilling the role of legal decision-maker, it is difficult to fully understand or contextualize the apparent moral premise that they were all on the same page regarding treatment. Are we to assume that the family's Persian identity necessarily entails a view that the female family members will defer to the male head of the family, or perhaps that even if there are family discussions happening behind the scenes that the male head of the family fully and sufficiently represents the views of the entire family to outsiders? Having cultural sensitivity does not mean that one should hold cultural stereotypes or fail to explore the unique nature of the family dynamics and relationships.

What Is the Ethical Issue That Needs to Be Resolved?

The role of ethics consultation is broad, from identifying and analyzing ethics concerns, facilitating communication, representing institutional policies, addressing knowledge gaps, integrating values into decision-making, and more. In this case, the focus of the meetings between care providers and the patient's family is on whether or not to provide CPR. The physician team seems to present a united front stating that the patient was not a candidate for further curative treatments, yet they also continue to offer those treatments and seem dismayed when the family chooses the treatments that are offered. Dr. Broukhim and Dr. Moore have specifically attempted to ensure that Mrs. Hamadani's children understand the ethical dimensions of the decisions that are being made, and Mrs. Hamadani's children have made it clear that they understand not only the clinical picture but also concerns about the patient's suffering. Weighing the information, the children have clearly communicated their decisions regarding treatment. Mr. Zadeh is consistent and clear that he wishes to pursue all available treatments "until her heart stops," (Finder 2018: 25), and "until the decision to act must be made" (Finder 2018: 31). Because the family is always at the bedside and thus available, it seems reasonable to assume they can fulfill their wish to make decisions only when decisions must be made, taking into account their mother's current clinical picture and the information provided by the clinical team. They have fulfilled their decision-making role by understanding the information presented to them, integrating their (and hopefully the patient's) values, and they have communicated their decisions regarding the clinical questions posed to them. There is not confusion about the clinical picture or what the family has decided and the team has concrete guidance on how to proceed. Finder points out that the case does not fall under the hospital's medically inappropriate treatment policy, and we are not presented with evidence the care being provided violates the patient's wishes or the standard of care. Finally, despite his reluctance, Dr. Broukhim appears willing to continue his care of the patient and follow the family's decisions. As a result, it seems that the issue of the patient's code status has been resolved, and the work that remains is helping the medical team understand and/or cope with the family's decisions.

I should note here that the impasse regarding code status may represent cultural differences in the meaning of time. Medical treatment plans at the end-of-life can be skewed toward anticipating what may happen and creating plans to address it. Forward-looking planning as a core value can be in opposition to a focus on the human interactions taking place in the moment and the desire to address decisions each in their own time. This is a tension between the desire to have time to prepare versus having time to spend interacting and expressing relationships. Certainly, we walk away from the narrative with an understanding that the family values spending time with their mother more than planning for her death.

Despite having an informed and clearly articulated plan of care, it is significant that the meetings in the narrative continue to focus on convincing the patient's children to make a different decision, rather than exploring the family's reasoning and goals for their mother. Changing the focus of conversations to create a better understanding of the family's reasons for their decisions may help care providers better accept having to act on a decision reflecting values that they do not appear to share. For example, while Dr. Broukhim may be prioritizing the minimization of perceived suffering, the patient's children may be prioritizing a different set of goals such as a duty to ensure they had fully explored every option for their mother or honoring their mother's wish to 'go down fighting.' In the same vein, discussions regarding their goals and what was motivating their reasoning process could also reveal powerful emotional states such as fear, guilt or grief which might be controlling their perceptions and choices.

Regardless, changing the focus of discussion to goals rather than procedures could help to create a more positive dialogue between all persons involved with the patient's care, even if the family does not change their mind regarding code status. A better understanding of the family's reasoning and motivations may also have helped the team better cope with or accept the family's decisions (the very point that Dr. Moore was pursuing when he was removed from the case).

A different issue represents another clear area of ethical concern. There are instances in the narrative where staff appear distressed during interactions with the patient's family, yet that distress is not explored in the narrative, nor are its potential solutions. Specifically, we are told "someone involved in her care—perhaps the consulting nephrologists or the ICU attending or the Social Worker" were concerned that Mrs. Hamadani was suffering (Finder 2018: 23). The perception that the patient is suffering is deeply concerning and deserving of further exploration. What do the persons involved mean by "suffering"? Were her symptoms poorly controlled, was she feeling depressed, or was she unsupported in pursuing her own goals? Was the source of the distress the perception that the family was poorly treating the staff who were caring for Mrs. Hamadani, or was it discomfort with the moral subjectivity that is inherent in end-of-life decisions? How are these issues being addressed by the Palliative Care service on this admission? These issues are clearly within the scope of the ethics consultation, yet we are not provided with an understanding of how suffering was being addressed or how such concerns were resolved. This may be a result of the hybrid assignment of ethics consultant duties, with Dr. Moore supporting the staff and other physicians and Finder supporting the family and working with Dr. Broukhim. In the end, the unresolved issues in the narrative regarding the staff's distress and perception that the patient was suffering seem to be clear ethical concerns that warrant the reasoned deliberation of the ethics consultant.

Scope of Ethics Consultation

"The Zadeh Scenario" presents several elements that raise questions about the scope of ethics consultation. Three such elements merit some explicit discussion: referrals, use of the electronic medical record to follow-up on patients, and the process of requesting an ethics consultation. In regards to referrals, during the initial ethics consultation 3 years ago, Dr. Moore solicited the involvement of a physician that would more closely align with the family's aggressive treatment goals: "In an effort to help this family, Steve was the one who had actually contacted Dr. Broukhim to see if he'd be willing to talk with Mr. Zadeh and his sisters" (Finder 2018: 22–3). This went beyond a mere recommendation regarding other available physicians which the family could choose or not choose to follow-up on. The consultant actually made the call himself based on his knowledge of Dr. Broukhim's reputation. Though it remains unclear how the recommendation came about and the process of consent that preceded the call, this action suggests pushing the bounds of clinical ethics consultation. One could be skeptical that the ethicist directly soliciting the new involvement of specific providers who best match the value-based goals of the patient/family is within the moral scope of the consultant's responsibility.

The use of the electronic medical record to track readmissions of patients who have previously been seen by the ethics consultation service shines a light on several questions: When does a consult end? Is follow-up to an ethics consultation part of continuity of care? Is the consultant part of the clinical team with a responsibility to the continuity of care? To be sure, the consultant is an actively engaged participant who serves a unique role as a facilitator and mediator in explicit discussions of values and beliefs which must be understood against a specific set of circumstances and relevant standards. As a practical endeavor, facilitating accountable and ethically justifiable solutions means that as the clinical picture changes, so too may the ethically justifiable solutions. The ethics consultation detailed here provides a tangible example of intense value-laden discussions occurring over the course of an ethics consult. It further illustrates the fact that complex issues rarely become less complex merely because a plan of action is undertaken.

In his work with the patient/family and the health care providers over past hospitalizations, Dr. Moore has elicited and attended to the values, beliefs and judgments embedded in the activities and decisions of the patient's hospitalizations. How and why the beliefs and judgments of the stakeholders change over time can be morally significant, and because it can be difficult to capture all of the nuance or breadth of discussions in medical record documentation, it is often times the ethics consultant who is the repository and voice of those moral experiences. As the clinical situation changes, decision-making may require a return to those previous discussions, which now require new interpretations or application.

This does not mean, however, that ethics consultants have a moral responsibility to act everywhere a moral issue requires clarification. To do so runs the risk of obfuscating the moral responsibility of other staff. However, the ethical justification that grounds actions and plans of care can atrophy over time in the face of nearly constant turnover in care providers and institutional processes designed more toward standardization than individualization. In this case, Dr. Moore's continued involvement provides a stable point of contact and preserves the critical historical knowledge of those previous conversations and stages of understanding. While an electronic medical record that flags previous patients seen by the service upon their readmission involves important issues of privacy and confidentiality, as long as the patient/family were both aware of the consultant's potential involvement and did not object, this model of follow-up may be a salutary, if not always feasible practice.

In regards to the process of requesting an ethics consultation, we are told that during admissions following the initial consultation, Dr. Moore was "informally" asked by various staff members to "formally" intervene. The language of 'informality' is worth noting. There are many ways that staff may experience moral moments while caring for patients. Some moral moments are experienced as a call to action while others may be experienced as self-reflection or moral distress. The ethics consultant can recognize, facilitate and affirm the complex emotions that may accompany these moments, but a line can and should be drawn between creating a safe space to discuss and examine moral feelings and a responsibility to follow-up and take action on issues uncovered during such discussions. Any person involved in the patient's care should have standing to call an ethics consult, but should do so within a formal process wherein the requestor takes responsibility for involving the ethics consultant, not just hope that the consultant will take the hint. A process of ethics consultation should lead to enhanced ethical understanding among the parties, but not rob stakeholders of their own ethical responsibility and moral agency.

Conclusion

In conclusion, "The Zadeh Scenario" offers many important insights regarding the activities inherent in the process of ethics consultation. Nonetheless, we see that an account of the clinical engagement of a consultant is ultimately not enough to provide a holistic account of the consultant's practice, or to discern the core moral considerations that emerge among the divergent standpoints. Furthermore, much of the information that is needed to both understand and assess the role of the consultant, the goals of consultation, and the broader societal and legal context in which ethics consultations occur lies outside the parameters of a particular case – no matter how detailed or beautifully told.

References

American Medical Association (2014) Code of medical ethics of the American Medical Association Council on ethical and judicial affairs: current opinions with annotations, 2014–2015 edition. American Medical Association, Chicago

Finder SG (2018) The Zadeh scenario. In: Finder SG, Bliton MJ (eds) Peer review, peer education, and modeling in the practice of clinical ethics consultation: the Zadeh project. Springer, Cham, pp 21–42

Ethics Consultation for Mrs. Hamadani – A Focus on Process

Anita J. Tarzian

Introduction

My appreciation for *process* in ethics consultation was taken up a notch after experiencing how much thought our neighbors to the North put into procedural elements of professional practice. In 2011, I was privileged to attend a meeting of Canada's "Practicing Healthcare Ethicists Exploring Professionalization" (PHEEP) group in Saint John, New Brunswick.[1] Much of that meeting was spent attending to how the newly-formed group would work together. While some of the Canadians bemoaned their commitment to *how* things are done as much as to *what* is accomplished, I remember making a "note to self" along the lines of: *Attending mindfully to the process of how health care ethics consultation is done is just as important as demonstrating that ethics consultants have requisite skills and knowledge.*

My work chairing the American Society for Bioethics and Humanities' (ASBH's) Core Competencies Update Task Force (Tarzian & the ASBH Core Competencies Update Task Force, 2013), and my membership on ASBH's Quality Attestation Presidential Task Force, left me with an appreciation for procedural standards in health care ethics consultation (HCEC). Decades ago, when new ethical dilemmas and uncertainties borne out of medical innovations emerged on the front lines of health care delivery, and bewildered clinicians looked for someone to help them sort through the various ethical questions that arose, identifying what specific steps those "helping" such clinicians should follow was not a priority. The focus was more aptly situated on the ethical analyses applied to address uncertainty about the

[1] Now the Canadian Association of Practicing Healthcare Ethicists – Association canadienne des éthiciens en soins de santé (CAPHE-ACESS).

A. J. Tarzian (✉)
University of Maryland School of Nursing; Program Coordinator, Maryland Healthcare Ethics Committee Network at UM Carey Law, Baltimore, MD, USA
e-mail: atarzian@comcast.net

S. G. Finder, M. J. Bliton (eds.), *Peer Review, Peer Education, and Modeling in the Practice of Clinical Ethics Consultation: The Zadeh Project*,
https://doi.org/10.1007/978-3-319-90955-4_5

right decision or course of action to take in particular situations. Decades later, in a new century, when ethics consultation is available in most U.S. hospitals and is legislated in some states, the landscape has changed. We now have a code of ethics for HCE consultants which, among other things,[2] obligates HCE consultants to "Be competent," to "Manage conflicts of interest and obligation," to "Contribute to the field," and to "Promote just health care within HCEC." Meeting these professional responsibilities requires active peer review. Toward that end, I'm grateful for the opportunity to provide my observations regarding Finder's involvement in the Hamadani ethics consultation.[3]

Was This an Ethics Consultation?

The first question is, did Finder provide an *ethics consultation, or* another ethics service in his role as health care ethics (HCE) consultant? The *Core Competencies for Healthcare Ethics Consultation* ("*Core Competencies*" ASBH 2011, p. 3) defines an ethics consultation as a "response to questions from patients, families, surrogates, health care professionals, or other involved parties who seek to resolve uncertainty or conflict regarding value-laden concerns that emerge in health care." HCE consultants can provide other services in addition to ethics consultation, such as ethics "coaching" and ethics education outside of what occurs during HCEC, overseeing an ethics consultation service, engaging in research or quality improvement initiatives, publishing scholarly work, mentoring other ethics consultants or interns, or providing proactive ethics services (Chidwick et al. 2010). It appears that not only was Finder's help solicited directly to address a question involving values conflicts, but Moore had also been asked to intervene by staff—both during this hospital stay and prior hospital stays—to help resolve perceived conflicts between Mrs. Hamadani's children and the staff members caring for her. Thus, I do think this falls under the definition of ethics consultation, which is relevant in how Finder's performance is evaluated.

[2] The code of ethics responsibility to "Respect privacy and maintain confidentiality" requires either modifying the details of published case summaries so that those involved cannot be recognized, or obtaining permission to publish the summary of a case in which those involved might be recognizable. I have confirmed that this standard has been met for the Hamadani case, and I appreciate the book editors' attention to meeting this professional standard.

[3] Just as an ethics case consultation requires collecting information from involved parties to identify relevant contextual issues related to the case, an analysis of the HCE consultant's performance in a given case consultation likewise requires having access to contextual details. Finder has provided a rich recounting of the facts surrounding Mrs. Hamadani's final hospital stay and conflicts that arose between Mrs. Hamadani's children and her health care providers. Yet, a caveat of this performance evaluation is that information was not gathered first-hand. For example, I did not review any of Finder's notes written about this ethics consultation, nor speak first-hand with any of the involved parties. Thus, what I can provide here is an analysis of Finder's performance as ethics consultant based solely on the information he provided.

Case Consultation or Something Else?

The next question is whether this constituted an ethics *case consultation,* i.e., an ethics consultation in which the HCE consultant interacts with a patient and/or the patient's family members. If the answer is "yes," then we would expect to see documentation of the HCEC in the patient's medical record. Other types of ethics consultations (referred to as "non-case consultations" in the *Core Competencies*) typically involve working solely with health care staff (e.g., helping staff debrief or process a difficult patient care situation, or helping them consider the ethical implications of a new institutional policy). Given Finder's interactions with Mrs. Hamadani's children, this seems aptly characterized as a case consultation. But there is a descriptive and a normative question here: *was* the consultation request handled as a case consultation, and *should it* have been handled as a case consultation?

Let's work backwards to consider Dr. Moore's involvement, since that influenced how Finder became involved. In a prior hospitalization, Dr. Moore responded to an ethics consultation request from a neurologist to address concerns that the Hamadani family was inappropriately requesting life-prolonging treatments for Mrs. Hamadani that increased her suffering without appreciably benefitting her. There appear to have been concerns about how the Hamadani children interacted with staff, and perhaps some concern with how decisions were being made for Mrs. Hamadani. The *Core Competencies* (2011) encourages each institution to have an identified process for how its ethics consultation service will handle HCEC requests. That way, consultations can be evaluated based on whether they meet institution-based standards (which should meet field-wide HCEC standards). Initially, the consultant should clarify the request. As stated in the *Core Competencies* (ASBH 2011: 12):

> Generally this requires considering the preliminary information received at the time of the request, confirming that the request is appropriate for ethics consultation, setting reasonable expectations with the requester about what the ethics consultant will and will not do, and developing an initial formulation of the ethics question(s) that will be addressed by the consultation.

Presumably, Dr. Moore confirmed that the staff member requesting the initial consultation preferred that Dr. Moore treat this as an ethics case consultation, which would involve Dr. Moore speaking directly with various stakeholders— including with Mrs. Hamadani (if able) and the Hamadani children—to gather information (alone if using a single-consultant model; in collaboration with other ethics consultants if using a duo or team model). This might have been followed by a meeting with staff (often first without and later with the Hamadani family), with Dr. Moore leading those meetings.

I think it would be appropriate to proceed with a case consultation approach if Dr. Moore believed this was the best way to meet the needs of those involved. Often, health care staff prefer such an approach because it frees up time they would otherwise have to spend communicating with various stakeholders, and they value the unbiased perspective of the ethics consultant(s). However, I also think it's valuable to offer options when they exist and to clarify the preferred role the ethics consultant is playing. For example, staff might value an opportunity to review with Dr. Moore how they have been communicating with the Hamadani family about goals of care and decision-making as her cancer spread and her disease progressed. The mentioned lack of anyone taking a lead in identifying what interventions, if any, were no longer appropriate to offer Mrs. Hamadani demonstrates a failure of leadership on the part of the attending physician that should be addressed. Dr. Moore could either offer to take on the traditional role of the ethics consultant facilitating communication across consulting services, or he could offer to work with the attending physician to identify better ways of ensuring that the staff are "all on the same page."

The difference here is mostly procedural, and I'll return to this when addressing Finder's involvement in the case. The point is that having a standard approach to ethics consultation does not mean that the ethics consultant must play the same role in each consultation—rather, the consultant should find out what the requestor wants help with and then clarify how the consultant proposes to help. For example, the ethics consultant could have offered to accompany staff when they met with members of the Hamadani family (alone or during care coordination meetings) to provide feedback on communication encounters. In this instance, rather than acting as "lead consultant" in facilitating a formal meeting with the patient/family and the health care staff, the ethics consultant would be playing the role of ethics expert by providing constructive feedback about how the staff are communicating with each other and with the Hamadani family. Or, if the central issue focused on the conflict over Mrs. Hamadani's resuscitation status, Finder may have played a mediation role. The importance is allowing for the role of the ethics consultant to match the needs of the requestor(s), and clarifying what role the ethics consultant is playing.

T'aarof as Ethics?

Finder wisely identified many cultural influences that complicated the Hamadani ethics consultation. I'm reminded of a medical Grand Rounds presentation I gave many years ago entitled, "Challenging the Golden Rule: The Influence of Culture in Healthcare Encounters." Along with other examples, I referenced the Persian concept of *T'aarof,* a ritual politeness code that governs behaviors between individuals of different hierarchies and imposes obligations to mitigate emotional distress by way of avoiding negative feelings through specific culturally-engrained social etiquette. An Iranian physician in the audience admitted to feeling overwhelmed by competing cultural and professional obligations when caring for his traditional Iranian patients. He asked me what he could do about this. It struck me that providing "culturally competent care" is a challenge not only when a clinician comes from a culture that is different from the patient's culture, but also when the clinician shares a culture with a patient that differs from mainstream U.S. medical culture. It's clear that this contributed substantially to the perceived conflicts between the Hamadani family and the staff caring for Mrs. Hamadani. What's less clear is the role that the ethics consultants played in addressing the ethical issues encountered by those involved.

The Role of the Ethics Consultant

It's a poignant note that Samir, Mrs. Hamadani's son, first thought to ask Finder for help after seeing the title "Director of Ethics" on his name badge. From the description of how the interactions between the Hamadani family and hospital staff unfolded, it's likely that Samir's understanding of "ethics" and Finder's role as an ethics consultant differed from other staff members' perceptions. Despite some of the Hamadani children being more acculturated to the U.S. than others, there are several examples provided indicating that *T'aarof* may have influenced their expectations and led them to perceive that hospital staff had breached culturally-embedded ethical norms of conduct, Dr. Broukhim notwithstanding. Finder aptly identifies several of these norms: being a good listener, showing an interest and spending time getting to know family members, not distracting family away from the patient's bedside, the youngest son avoiding thinking about his mother's death to remain "strong" for his older sisters, and not focusing on what *won't* be done at the moment of death but on what it means to respect and care for one's mother leading up to and at the moment of her death.

Let's assume that Samir's expectation in asking for Finder's help was to reconcile a perceived breach of good conduct on the part of Dr. Moore. Is this a valid request for ethics consultation? While lodging a complaint about a "bad actor" often involves referring the requestor to the appropriate supervisor for follow up, in this case, I would argue that Samir's request is appropriate for ethics consultation, given the prior history and complex components of the case. Finder appropriately addresses the question of who should respond to this consult by concluding that one shouldn't force family members to talk with ethics consultants they don't want to talk to, and since Samir requested that Dr. Moore no longer speak with him or his sisters, Finder takes over Dr. Moore's role as the ethics consultant on this case. As Director of Ethics and thus Dr. Moore's supervisor, this simplifies Finder's decision to take over the case (since he presumably has the authority to do this).

Finder writes down some notes about his conversation with Samir, he reviews Mrs. Hamadani's chart, he talks with the intensive care unit (ICU) staff, and he meets with Dr. Broukhim. This is a good beginning. From this point on, however, there is ambiguity in several procedural aspects of how this consultation was handled. First, it wasn't entirely clear how limits on Dr. Moore's involvement would be communicated to other staff, as Finder stated to Moore: "I think it's OK if you want to keep talking with Broukhim since you've been helping him as much as anything. But really try not to put yourself in a position that the family might misperceive as your still being involved with them. I'll take over that" (Finder 2018: 28). Second, it's not clear that Finder has clarified what role he will play in this case. When meeting with Dr. Broukhim and Mrs. Hamadani's children, it's Dr. Broukhim who leads the discussion, leaving Finder to ponder how he should contribute. It's Dr. Broukhim who suggests, in his chart notes, the kind of assistance Finder can offer, including to "provide support" to the family, to "delineate ethical issues" involving Mrs. Hamadani's care, "not to persuade or to be abrasive" but "just to provide more care for them in these trying times" (Finder 2018: 30). Dr. Broukhim explains to Samir that the meeting with Finder "is not about Dr. Moore or Ethics Consultation but only about his mother" (Finder 2018: 30). Finder wonders if Dr. Broukhim is looking for "reassurance that he was helping Mrs. Hamadani's children come to accept that he had few to no options left to provide for their mother" (Finder 2018: 34).

It would have been helpful if Finder had clarified his role with Dr. Broukhim before the first meeting with Samir, Nadira, and Farzana, as Finder admits: "I wasn't sure if I was there to help Dr. Broukhim or to facilitate a conversation, or both, or just to bear witness…" (Finder 2018: 38). Finder ultimately suggests that Dr. Broukhim play the role of communication broker, telling Samir, Nadira and Farzana that "all the communication about what's going to be done for your mother [can] flow through him" to keep everyone "on the same page" so that "what one person says is not misunderstood or confused by what others say or mean or intend" (Finder 2018: 41). Does Finder mean that he will assist Dr. Broukhim in communicating with other members of the treatment team? It's unclear. He goes on to tell Mrs. Hamadani's children that the "real issue" is making sure that they understand what's going on and that their "expectations match" to avoid the problem of not being "prepared for what's staring us in the face." Again, it's unclear what this means, exactly. Who really *is* in charge, and how is Finder helping resolve this ambiguity?

Influence of Various Cultural Orientations

Just as Mrs. Hamadani and her children come from a particular cultural orientation, members of her treatment team come from their own personal and professional cultural orientations. Dr. Broukhim's orientation is influenced both by his professional training and his Persian roots. He spends many hours with his patients, referring to his "respect" and "devotion" toward his patients and their family members, writing detailed notes in their charts, and offering oncology treatments that some of his colleagues believe go "too far" in promoting "false hopes." Finder hints at the professional cultural norms in Western acute care and oncology settings. For example, it's clear that most of the staff caring for Mrs. Hamadani believed that when metastatic cancer is inoperable and advanced, ICU-level care and related interventions (such as intubation and ventilation, renal dialysis, and cardio-pulmonary resuscitation attempts) cause more harm than benefit and in some instances should not be offered. There are several references to staff focusing on interventions that should be withheld or withdrawn, as evident in Dr. Moore's advice to Finder: "I'd just warn you that they may be using you, to avoid what we'd already agreed upon in terms of talking about why they want to code her and have the feeding tube and whatever other aggressive interventions that may be available" (Finder 2018: 28).

While Finder recognizes these cultural differences in his write-up of "The Zadeh Scenario," it's unclear whether or how he addressed these conflicts in his role as the ethics consultant. It seems even Dr. Broukim questions whether he goes too far in what he offers to his patients. For example, he asks Finder whether dialysis would be reasonable for Mrs. Hamadani. Finder replies that while there are those who would consider dialysis in this case to be "a bad use of a limited resource" and "a prime example of why our healthcare system is in the state it's in and why we need reform," that if the goal of care is to give Mrs. Hamadani "a few more days," a few rounds of dialysis could help (Finder 2018: 35). Is this guidance sufficient to address the ethical conflicts this case presents?

Mixed Messages

Given that Mrs. Hamadani cannot communicate her wishes and there's no mention of an advance directive, medical decision-making is shared between her children and the attending physician (it's implied that Dr. Broukhim is the attending physician; the ICU attending's role is unclear). Finder assumes that Mrs. Hamadani's children are making choices based on what she would have wanted and/or on her best interests. What choices are available to them depends on the medical standard of care. This is where additional ambiguity clouds the ethics consultant's role. What medical interventions should be available to Mrs. Hamadani—and patients as sick as her—is an open question. The staff believed Mrs. Hamadani's children were making bad decisions and causing their mother to suffer. Finder uses the word "futile" to describe how staff felt about the use of aggressive life-prolonging interventions for Mrs. Hamadani (Finder 2018: 23). But he doesn't address *which* proposed interventions, if any, might actually fall into that category. The physicians involved in this case appear to disagree about what medical interventions were appropriate for Mrs. Hamadani. For example, Dr. Smith and Dr. Nadouri do not consider dialysis to be helpful in achieving "long-term goals" (Finder 2018: 31).

The role of the ethics consultant in such a case should be to help reduce this ambiguity by facilitating communication and educating those involved about standards for decision-making and for resolving conflicts. For example, White and Wicclair (2012) proposed three categories of medical interventions: generally accepted, generally unaccepted, and a middle category comprising the "grey zone." Grey zone interventions are often at the center of ethics consultations. White and Wicclair proposed that within the grey zone, clinicians should identify "medically inadvisable" interventions that should be withheld or withdrawn and should use a fair process for resolving disagreements. These are interventions that might accomplish an effect that a patient or family member desires, but that could be withheld based on the following ethical justifications: (1) they are unlikely to achieve their intended goal, (2) the goal they are intended to achieve is of controversial value, or (3) they are not cost-effective. This is consistent with a more recent policy statement on "potentially inappropriate treatment" developed by the Society of Critical Care Medicine's ethics committee (Kon et al. 2016).

Dr. Broukhim recommends that Mrs. Hamadani forego cardio-pulmonary resuscitation (CPR) attempts, as this "will not change the inevitability that awaits her" and "will likely cause her harm" (Finder 2018: 40). He communicates this to her children, but also tells them that if they wished their mother to be "coded" then he would "support them" (Finder 2018: 40). This is a mixed message. Similarly, he provides the children with vivid depictions of their mother's deteriorating physical status and impending death, but then reassures them that he is not trying to "change their mind about what to do" or getting them to "say that they should withhold additional interventions or even withdraw any of the support currently being provided" (Finder 2018: 39). Perhaps like the Iranian physician in my Grand Rounds presentation, Dr. Broukhim struggles with what *T'aarof* demands in these situations. It clearly results in confusion regarding what interventions Mrs. Hamadani can receive. It's also unclear to the Hamadani children and perhaps to Dr. Broukhim himself that their decision-making is shared, but that ultimately, the attending physician writes medical orders, as Mrs. Hamadani's children believe they can decide themselves whether their mother is intubated or whether CPR is attempted (when in fact these are *medical* orders). Why didn't Finder point out these contradictions to Dr. Broukhim? Why not assemble the treatment team and facilitate a discussion about how judgments should be made about which treatments are considered medically inappropriate, and where to draw the line with what should be offered to Mrs. Hamadani and similarly situated patients?

Ambiguity Regarding Ethically Appropriate Interventions

Finder's involvement with Mrs. Hamadani originated from Samir's dissatisfaction that Dr. Moore and the staff were over-focusing on a Do-Not-Resuscitate (DNR) order for his mother. Finder alludes to—but doesn't explicitly articulate—the actual ethical issues he identifies after talking to all those involved. Staff are angry and resentful toward Mrs. Hamadani's children for making their mother suffer and for being overly demanding and at times intimidating; some are upset with Dr. Broukhim and Dr. Spector for offering interventions that appeared to meet White and Wicclair's definition of "medically inadvisable." This contributes to the conflict between Mrs. Hamadani's children and the treatment team, as evidenced by Samir exclaiming: "I do not need to hear 'we do not want your mother to suffer.' What I want is for my mother to be taken care of, and when the time comes to make a decision, my sisters and I will decide, and we will do what is best for our mother" (Finder 2018: 41).

The difficulty identifying which "grey zone" interventions qualify as "medically inadvisable" rests on judgments about which goals for Mrs. Hamadani are of "controversial value." The placement of a G-tube or naso-gastric tube is easier to classify as inadvisable for someone so close to death. Dialysis is a bit more difficult. A clinical practice guideline from the Renal Physicians Association (RPA 2010) recommends that dialysis not be provided to patients like Mrs. Hamadani who are near death from non-renal causes. Yet, the contested ICU transfer, blood pressure stabilizers, Bi-pap mask, and renal dialysis were implemented to achieve a goal of improving Mrs. Hamadani's mental status such that she could interact with her children one last time. Is this a worthwhile goal? Dr. Broukhim surmises: "it's not unreasonable to see if we can wake her up and give them a chance to have a little bit of final time together. She's been a real fighter all along, and they've been so involved in her care, I think I owe them this" (Finder 2018: 35). One may argue that this is an ethically justifiable goal, particularly given the likelihood that Dr. Broukhim has led Mrs. Hamadani's children to believe that her "fighting" to live is of value and something they should encourage. Dr. Broukhim would not be the first oncologist to interpret success as keeping his patients alive, while overlooking the value (and duty) of effectively preparing patients and their loved ones for death (hence, Samir's extreme reaction to the mention of hospice). He also would not be the first oncologist who needs support accepting his own patient's death and guidance in how to help families do the same (Graham 2013).

What's missing is a strategy for determining how these decisions are made in a way that minimizes regrets for the survivors, meets fairness criteria, and addresses the moral residue and distress of the staff. Mrs. Hamadani's children have asked that they speak with no other doctor but Dr. Broukhim— an unrealistic expectation, and perhaps one that Dr. Broukhim himself might have appreciated being liberated from with Finder's help. Nurses are refusing to care for Mrs. Hamadani. Samir "fires" the neurologist for mentioning hospice and Dr. Moore for talking about resuscitation status. These dynamics bode poorly for providing effective end-of-life care—either to Mrs. Hamadani or to others who are subject to the same staff communication breakdowns. Being a good listener is necessary—but not sufficient—for being an effective ethics consultant.

Conclusion

Despite the several potential shortcomings outlined above regarding how Finder handled the Hamadani case consultation, all was not lost. Just as an ounce of prevention is worth a pound of cure, a pound of active listening breeds ample good will. Finder facilitated good communication with Mrs. Hamadani's children and with Dr. Broukhim. He realized that discussing Mrs. Hamadani's resuscitation status or dialysis with Samir, Nadira or Farzana would only thwart future communication with them, so he simply listened. He picked up on the importance of spending time with them and asking them about their family. As far as his involvement with Samir, Nadira, Farzana, and Dr. Broukhim goes, this may fit within what I call a "mosaic" approach: even if parts are missing, there's enough there to see the whole picture. That is, even if Mrs. Hamadani's care was challenged by conflicting opinions and staff resentment, she died in a way that was consistent with how her family wished for her to be treated. Presumably, Samir, Nadira, and Farzana felt supported in the end.

It's unclear, however, whether the rest of the staff involved in this case felt supported by Finder's involvement. I wonder what would have happened if Finder had met with the treatment team after his initial involvement and facilitated a discussion about Mrs. Hamadani's care, her children's behavior, Iranian culture, and standards for judging interventions as "medically inadvisable." That way, a plan could have been constructed for how to provide respectful end-of-life care to Mrs. Hamadani without crossing ethical, professional, and emotional boundaries. Sometimes staff angst is grounded in frustration about the lack of consensus on where boundary lines are drawn, and poor communication about short- and long-term goals of care for a particular patient. The example of Mrs. Hamadani remaining a "full code" is a good one. Writing a DNR order over Samir's and Farzana's objections would have caused them distress and may have complicated their grieving. At the same time, the thought of having to attempt CPR for Mrs. Hamadani likely exacerbated the staff's distress. Here we have a classic conflict over positions. Could there be common interests underlying these competing positions? This is clearly the realm of the ethics consultant, but I didn't see where these ethics facilitation skills were applied to this case.

References

American Society for Bioethics and Humanities (2011) Core competencies for healthcare ethics consultation, 2nd edn. American Society for Bioethics and Humanities, Glenview

Chidwick P, Bell J, Connolly E, Couglin MD, Frolic A, Hardingham L, Zlotnik SR (2010) Exploring a model role description for ethicists. HEC Forum 22(1):31–40

Finder SG (2018) The Zadeh scenario. In: Finder SG, Bliton MJ (eds) Peer review, peer education, and modeling in the practice of clinical ethics consultation: the Zadeh project. Springer, Cham, pp 21–42

Graham J (2013) When the doctor disappears. The New York Times. Available at: http://newoldage.blogs.nytimes.com/2013/11/14/when-the-doctor-disappears/?_r=0. Last accessed 2 Nov 2014

Kon, A. et al. (2016). Defining futile and potentially inappropriate interventions: A Policy statement from the Society of Critical Care Medicine Ethics Committee. Crit Care Med, 44, 1769–17.

Renal Physicians Association (2010) Shared decision-making in the appropriate initiation of and withdrawal from dialysis, 2nd edn. Clinical Practice Guideline. Renal RPA, Rockville

Tarzian AJ, The ASBH Core Competencies Update Task Force (2013) Health care ethics consultation: an update on core competencies and emerging standards. AJOB 13(2):3–13

White DB, Wicclair M (2012) Limits on clinicians' discretion to unilaterally refuse treatment. Am J Crit Care 21(5):361–364

Ethics Consultation, Professional Praxis, and What it Means to Be a "Consultant"

James A. Hynds

Introduction

The situation described by Finder in "The Zadeh Scenario" is a very familiar one to those of us who work as ethicists in United States hospitals. The outcome he records, however, is unusually benign; indeed, and unfortunately, in many US hospitals the ultimately unresolved/unmediated conflict he describes would almost certainly result in the patient's being subjected to futile attempts at life-prolongation and resuscitation. In this sense, the outcome of this ethics consultation might be considered "good" insofar as it did not result in such futile attempts. But that sense of "good" is fleeting given other concerns which serve as the focus of this chapter.

Specifically, what follows is a constructive critique of how Finder, and Finder's colleague Moore, discharged their responsibilities as clinical ethics consultants in the situation Finder so carefully describes. In the course of offering this critique, I will necessary advance my own views about what ought to be involved in good ethics consultation. Indeed, let me begin my observations by doing that quite explicitly, by proposing a definition of what clinical ethics consultation (CEC) is. Although there is much to criticize in the American Society of Bioethics and the Humanities understanding of ethics consultation (Hynds 2013), their definition of the practice is, on the whole, sound:

> CEC consists in helping, upon request, the consult requester to identify, analysis and, where appropriate, resolve values uncertainty or conflict which arises in the context of providing medical care to a particular patient. The ultimate goal of the consult is to help the requester determine if, how and why a certain course of action should or should not be undertaken, based upon having identified, analyzed and, if possible, resolved the relevant values uncertainty or conflict which prompted the consult request. (ASBH 2011: 2)

J. A. Hynds (✉)
UCLA Health Ethics Center, Medicine, David Geffen School of Medicine,
University of California Los Angeles, Los Angeles, CA, USA
e-mail: JHynds@mednet.ucla.edu

S. G. Finder, M. J. Bliton (eds.), *Peer Review, Peer Education, and Modeling in the Practice of Clinical Ethics Consultation: The Zadeh Project*,
https://doi.org/10.1007/978-3-319-90955-4_6

In light of this understanding of the nature and goals of ethics consultation, upon which I attempt to base my own professional praxis, and although there is much to admire and emulate in the manner in which both Finder and Moore consulted in the situation Finder describes via "The Zadeh Scenario," I believe there are certain aspects of both Finder's and Moore's interactions with the staff, patient, family, and with each other that were highly problematic when evaluated in terms of their professional propriety. The discussion that follows focuses almost exclusively on these problematic aspects of their practice.

"Upon Request"

Clinical ethics consultants are, first and foremost, clinical *consultants*. Their involvement in a case presupposes that they have been invited to become involved by another person or group of persons. Only 'upon request' do ethics consultants participate *as* consultants in the care of patients. Accordingly, ethics consultants must not "self-authorize" their involvement. To do so suggests, *inter alia*, that clinical ethics consultation has a quasi-policing function: enforcing the compliance of other clinicians with some pre-existing mandatory standard of ethical behavior. Such a role has been rejected in principle (rightly, I believe) by the majority of those engaged in clinical ethics and the professional bodies that represent them (ASBH 2011: 4). Practically speaking, it is also the case that unsolicited involvement of an ethics consultant usually gives rise to a perception on the part of either the patient/family or the healthcare providers of being investigated and of being subtly (or not so subtly) pressured or even persecuted by the ethics consultant – hardly a perception likely to foster constructive relationships! It is a symptom of what ASBH calls the "authoritarian approach" to consultation (ASBH 2011: 6).

Proactivity and Continuity-of-Care

The fact that ethics consultants are *consultants* (i.e. require to be requested by another to legitimate involvement in a case) certainly poses problems for the ethics consultant who wants to ensure continuity of service over multiple hospital admissions (assuming that the same ethical uncertainties or conflicts persist) or who wants to be otherwise as proactive as possible in their consulting role. Finder and Moore, as the ethics consultants in this case, do clearly seem to be interested in continuity and pro-activity. But do they go about it in the right way?

Undoubtedly, Moore was initially consulted by the patient's neurologist (albeit after he had been dismissed from the patient's care) and latter he was consulted by

Dr. Broukhim. It is less clear, however, that Moore's involvement during the intervening hospitalizations was based on his having been formally consulted by anyone seeking his professional help. This fact may explain the rather unstructured nature of his involvement at that time, which is variously characterized as "stopping by" "checking in" or "simply following along." The lack of a formal consult request is problematic in itself and on account of the resultant sporadic nature of his interactions with clinicians and the family. 'Who was he trying to help?' may be legitimately ask.

How, then, should an ethics consultant handle multiple admissions of a patient for whom ethics consultation was requested at one point but not at those subsequent points of admission – and during those subsequent admissions may involve parties not involved in the initial consult request or non-involvement of the initial requesters? Similarly, what is the most appropriate way to manage a clinical ethics consultation that has "unfinished elements" at the time of the patient's discharge? And behind these two questions is a more fundamental issue: are pro-activity, continuity of service, and resolution/closure important values to be pursued in ethics consultation? I believe that they are. However, there are good and bad ways to go about achieving these ends.

One laudable way is to place a final summative ethics note in the patient's chart at or before the time of discharge. Such a note can include the ethics consultant's activities to date (including recommendations for current and reasonably foreseeable future ethical issues) and an offer to be available for re-consult at a future time, upon request, if that would be thought helpful by whoever assumes the care of the patient in subsequent re-admissions. Placing this type of summative ethics notes where it is most likely to be seen by subsequent health care providers – for instance, in an electronic medical record system's 'goals of care' tab with other notes which take a more global perspective on the management of the patient's healthcare – may be particularly useful, especially if the expectation in a health care system is that a new attending physician will read these notes immediately upon the re-admission of a patient. It is an excellent way to alert a physician to an ethics consultant's prior involvement in the care of the patient and to the possibility of re-engaging the clinical ethics consultation service if one so chooses.

Another more active – and possibly more aggressive – approach to maximize the possibility of ethics consultation continuity is for the ethics consultant to directly contact the new care team upon a patient's readmission in order to inform the team of past clinical ethics consultation involvement and to let them know that the ethics consultation service remains available should they wish to utilize it. This approach presupposes that the ethics consultant has an efficient notification system for when a patient is readmitted. But beyond that, other more aggressive attempts to ensure continuity is inappropriately intrusive; requiring re-engagement of the ethics consultation service, for example, is never appropriate (mandatory consultation, after all, is surely a contradiction in terms).

The Subjectivity of Consult Concerns

In addition to concerns about a lack of 'alter-authorization' to legitimate continuing ethics consultation, self-authorization is also problematic because new players (for want of a better expression) may not in fact have any ethical concerns regarding the current situation, or may have entirely different (perhaps even directly contradictory) ethical concerns from those of the initial consulter and/or the ethics consultant, even if there has been no material change in the patient's circumstances. Indeed, there is something intrinsically concerning about ethics consultants having ethical concerns of their own upon which they follow-up; it may not even be appropriate for an ethics consultant to decide that there 'is' an ethical issue that requires to be addressed. Clinical ethics consultation exists to help other people deal with issues that cause *them* ethical concern. The role of ethics consultation is not, therefore, to objectify those ethical concerns and then adopt them.

For all the above reasons, it is unwise for an ethics consultant simply to re-insert oneself into a formerly problematic situation simply because a patient for whom ethics consultation was provided previously is subsequently readmitted and, from the ethics consultant's perspective, the patient's circumstances still or again appear to be ethically challenging. But this appears to be exactly what Moore did – on several occasions – such that, when eventually asked formally to become re-involved, Mrs. Hamadani's children are, not surprisingly, upset; this leads them to reach out to Finder. Before turning to whether Finder's response to this was appropriate, a more basic question must be addressed.

Who May Call for a Consult?

If involvement of a clinical ethics consultant is not to originate in the ethics consultant's perspective of a clinical situation, who may legitimately request and be offered ethics consultation? Generally, there is agreement among ethics consultants that the right to ethics consultation, even although it is a clinical consult, is not limited exclusively to the patient's attending physician, as is generally the case with other clinical consults (ASBH 2011: 11). And in the case under discussion, a number of persons with different roles in the care of the patient either formally or informally appear to have requested ethics consultation.

The first requester for ethics consultation for this patient was the patient's former neurologist – "former" because at the time of his request, we are told, he was no longer actively involved in the patient's care, having just been fired by the family (indeed, this fact seems to have prompted him to request involvement of the clinical ethics consultation service in the first place). The question is what justifiable limits, if any, can and should be placed on access to ethics consultation for the sake of consulting in regard to the specific care of a specific patient? This is not an easy question to answer in a definitive way.

Access to ethics consultation should not simply be available to everyone, *simplex*. Rather, an appropriate requester (who may indeed occupy any position within the hospital, or none) must nevertheless demonstrate some degree of 'moral proximity' to ethical concerns that prompted the request. They must, in some sense, have a moral stake in the outcome of the ethics consultation: their own rights, responsibilities or legitimate interests must be significantly affected. This is something analogous to the idea of 'legal standing' which is used to determine if a prospective litigant has sufficient legal proximity to raise an action in Court. Whether the requester in fact demonstrates the necessary moral proximity is a matter of fact to be determined by the ethics consultant in exercise of his or her professional judgment. Determining moral proximity, in other words, is to be part of the ethics consultant's expertise. In relation to medical, nursing, and other staff involved in the care of a patient, it may well be that the requester either be or recently have been actively involved in the patient's care. The existence of clinical ethics consultation services in an institution must not be a blank check for unfettered good samaritanism.

Ethics Consultation: A Structure Engagement with the Issues

In regard to other formal (or process-oriented) deficiencies of Finder and Moore's consulting style, the seemingly unstructured or semi-structured way, at critical junctures in the process, which both consultants chose to engage the various issues/participants, is striking. On the part of Finder, this also appears to have been purposeful. Two examples of the seemingly unstructured or semi-structured process utilized by Finder and Moore stand out.

First, at no point in the extended involvement of Moore and then Finder with Mrs. Hamadani's situation was an interdisciplinary meeting suggested by Moore or Finder. The primary purpose of such a meeting would have been to ascertain directly from those with an interest (i.e. having moral proximity) if there was unanimity or at least a broad consensus among them concerning what the ethically appropriate course of action was with regard to Mrs. Hamadani's care, what that consensus was and, most importantly, why they thought it was the right thing to do *morally*. For many who provide ethics consultation, such a meeting is part of their being willing to consult in a case of this sort.

In addition to the above stated goals, such a meeting also allows clinicians with very different ethical perspectives and proposed solutions to share these and to receive feedback from their colleagues. Without such a forum, misunderstandings multiply and unspoken resentments can grow among team members. If a broad consensus does in fact exist among the clinicians (which is very often the case), that fact should be made clear to the family by having all the key players attend key meetings with them. This way of approaching things has the important benefit of minimizing the opportunities for 'splitting' that frequently characterizes family interactions with multiple clinicians.

In the case of Mrs. Hamadani's care, the momentum was (almost inevitably) in the opposite direction. Instead of bringing together the various interested parties, and seeking to establish if there was a consensus and what principled compromises, if any, could be made to achieve one, a process of fragmentation and exclusion seems to have occurred which appears to have been at very least tolerated, if not intentionally encouraged.

Second is the way in which Finder and Moore preferred to interact with Mrs. Hamadani's family. Throughout the narrative, both consultants meet with or talk to the family on multiple occasions alone, i.e., without the involvement of the consult requester or other persons having an interest in the resolution of the case. This is not to suggest that meeting one-on-one with a patient or the patient's family is never appropriate. Rather, the point is that the effectiveness of the ethics consultation process is always enhanced if interventions are kept to a minimum and all main participants in the situation are generally present. With regard to the frequency of ethics consultants' interaction with patients or families, the rationale for keeping interventions to a necessary minimum is to reduce the intrusive nature of the clinical ethics consultation process, respecting the need of the family to focus on their loved whose death (in this particular case) is relatively close and hence their opportunity to spend time with their loved one limited. Frequent interaction distracts from this and justly causes resentment. Moreover, constant meeting with the family has the appearance of being coercive, may be experienced as such, and may be undertaken by those who see their role (inappropriately, it must be added) as persuading the family to accept the ethical superiority of some particular plan of care the ethics consultant or the ethics consultation-requesting team happen to favor.

Involving as many of the interested parties as is reasonably practicable is also important since a central goal of ethics consultation is to seek to resolve conflict among these very persons. The mediating role of the ethics consultant is more easily exercised when everyone is sitting down at the same table. "Shuttle diplomacy" is generally unhelpful, except in situations where relationships have irretrievably broken down. Often ethical conflict is in fact the result of either poor or insufficient communication. This is more easily identified as a problem and resolved when the ethics consultant can directly observe how the parties are communicating or failing to communicate with each other. Meeting together also reduces the risks of "splitting" which often happens in these situations.

Whether as a non-clinician or a clinician who is not serving in that clinical role for the given patient, the ethics consultant also benefits from having the patient's physician(s) in attendance when meeting families in order to help the ethics consultant understand and address concerns arising from the specific clinical situation at that time. In the absence of the physician, the ethics consultant is likely to incorrectly state the clinical case or delay further discussion while re-consulting the physicians to bring the ethics consultant up to date with current clinical circumstances. Meeting the family with the physician in attendance (and ideally with the primary physician leading the meeting) also prevents the family from attempting to exclude input from the ethics consultant. The physician is entitled to invite whomsoever he feels will help him manage his patient appropriately – and this includes consulting with an ethics consultant.

Another deficiency of the process Finder's reporting presents concerns the failure to reference, discuss or invoke relevant hospital policy. At one point in the narrative, Finder mentions the fact that his institution has what is commonly known as a "futility policy" (Finder 2018: 23). Notwithstanding the existence of such a policy, it seemed to have played little if any explicit part in how the case was managed. But the policy and the processes for conflict resolution it contains (including the possibility of a clinical ethics consultation) should help frame and structure the whole process of engagement, including the ethics consultation itself.

Professional Collegiality

Consider now a final problematic aspect of this case in relation to the formalities of the ethics consultation process. Specifically, attention must be turned toward the appropriateness of the interactions between Finder and Moore following – and apparently in response to – Mrs. Hamadani's family's request that Moore be relieved of his duties by Finder in the latter's capacity as 'Director' of the clinical ethics consultation service.

In coming to a judgment about whether it was appropriate for Finder to replace Moore (which he seems effectively to have done), the following question must be asked: What is the appropriate way to understand the relationship between Finder and Moore (and by extension, the relationship between directors of clinical ethics consultation services in general and the ethics consultants who discharge the consulting function of those services the directors direct)? Is it a hierarchic relationship? Does a consultant *qua* consultant work "under" the director, and at his direction as Mrs. Hamadani's family appear to believe, and as Finder's replacement of Moore at the family's request might reasonably be interpreted to confirm? And even if Moore is related to Finder in such a way, was it appropriate for Moore to be replaced as the consultant at the request of the family in the particular way that Finder ultimately did? These issues are organizational issues and at the same time ethical issues. We need to remember that ethics consultation itself has its own organizational ethics issues to address – issues which have to date attracted too little attention, especially when considered in terms of the professionalization of our discipline.

If clinical ethics consultation is a truly professional undertaking,[1] and if the individual ethics consultant is a professional practitioner in the full sense of that term (both of which are loaded questions) then it is highly problematic to characterize the relationship Finder and Moore are in as one in which the latter, in the discharge of

[1] Much of the debate on whether ethics consultation can properly be understood as a professional undertaking is focused on the question of whether clinical ethicists possess ethics expertise. An excellent introduction to the question is provided by Rasmussen (2016).

his consulting responsibilities, works “under” the former. Having been consulted by a legitimate requester, Moore assumes the responsibilities and, in consequence, the rights associated with his professional status, the core of which is the exercise of professional judgment. It is in the exercise of individual judgment (having perhaps freely sought advice from colleagues) that professionalism consists and for which a professional is properly held accountable. If the consultant is a professional, he must be free from undue influence or, worse, interference in the exercise and execution of his professional judgment, including direct interference from the director of the ethics consultation service.

In this regard, an ethics consultant should enjoy the same type of relationship with his director as other professional members of the staff. The most apt clinical analogy to the proper relationship between a director of a clinical ethics consultation service and an individual ethics consultant is that between the director of a particular medical service (e.g. the Director of an ICU) and individual attending physicians who care for patients in the unit managed by the director. It would clearly be inappropriate in almost every circumstances for the unit director to attempt to involve himself directly in the medical care of a particular patient without the knowledge and consent of the attending physician.

One can, of course, envision certain circumstances where a director may feel the need (and indeed may have the responsibility) to intervene in a particular case, on his own initiative or upon the request of a third party. The justification for so doing in a professional model, however, would be based presumably on a well-founded concern on the part of the director regarding either the competence of the consultant or accusations of professionally inappropriate behaviors. In other words, the director’s intervention would be justified, and can only be justified, precisely in terms of safeguarding the professional nature of the service the consultant, as a member of the department, is legitimately expected to provide. Neither justification, however, would appear to have been invoked (explicitly or implicitly) by Finder when he intervened (interfered?) in Moore’s serving as an ethics consultant for Mrs. Hamadani’s situation.

Having said all this, it is not inappropriate for a director to inform a consultant that a patient or a family has asked him to relieve the consultant of his consulting responsibilities. He may ask the consultant if he wants to withdraw from the case on account of the family request, and may offer to replace him. He may even recommend (strongly) that the consultant step aside to be replaced by another consultant (including himself if he ordinarily fulfills that role) who is more likely to achieve the ends of that ethics consultation. But short of evidence of negligence or improper behavior on the part of the ethics consultant, the director should not, as a general rule, require an ethics consultant to withdraw from a case or worse yet, become actively involved in the case without the ethics consultant’s knowledge or consent. To do otherwise is to cultivate a non-professional profile of the service he directs and of those who offer it.

Nor is it clear that such an intervention (i.e. replacing the consultant) would as a matter of fact relieve a consultant of the (legal) responsibilities they had undertaken by entering into a consulting relationship. If this is the case, it would appear to be a highly imprudent move on the part of a consultant to allow another individual (including the director) to effectively take over operational control of a consultation for which the consultant continues to have some degree of on-going professional responsibility. But this seems to be exactly what transpires between Finder and Moore.

Similar dangers exist where a director may from time to time informally involve himself in the consultations of his colleagues, a habit more likely to be found where curbside consultation is tolerated or encouraged in a department. In the same vein, a director should probably avoid giving informal advice to colleagues about what should be done in a case lest the advice be interpreted by the consultant as an instruction to give effect to the director's recommendations. Ethics consultants would do well to remember that 'superior orders' are unlikely to be accepted as a defense to a claim for professional negligence or misconduct.

A different evaluation of Finder's intervention in this case may very well have been reached if there was some evidence to suggests that his department was differently structured or staffed. If, for example, Finder was the only professional ethicist in the department and/or Moore was very significantly less professionally qualified or expert than Finder, it may have been appropriate for the former to interpose himself in the way he appears to have done. The obvious example of such an occurrence would be in circumstances where team consultation is the norm in an institution and where the level of ethics competence often varies among members of the team.[2] In those circumstances, it could be appropriate for the director on his own initiative or upon request of another to either supplement or replace the initial ethics consultant(s). A professionally adequate response to the challenges involved in a particular ethics consultation might demand a higher level of expertise and/or experience than the initial ethics consultant happens to possess. In this light, it is regrettable that team consultation as it is envisaged by ASBH continues to be acceptable: it is hard to see how it is compatible with the evolving understanding of clinical ethics consultation as a professional practice.

Be that as it may, if the possibility exists within a department, for whatever reason, of an ethics consultant being replaced by the director of the service, the circumstances in which it may or will happen should be clearly delineated and known to the consultant in advance. Similarly, if a decision is made by the director to jointly consult with an ethics consultant, then it is important to delineate the respective roles, responsibilities, and rights of each of the professionals involved.

Nothing in this section should be taken to disparage the propriety of an ethics consultation requester asking for and obtaining a second ethics opinion. Indeed, in some circumstances, it might be appropriate for an ethics consultant himself to suggest that the requester formally seek a second ethics opinion. The possibility of

[2] ASBH accepts that ethics consultation may be carried out by 'teams', the members of which need only collectively embody the full range of core competencies. The Society explicitly talks about individual team members who, possessing basic competence, are authorized to perform ethics consultation *"only under the supervision of a more senior member of the HCEC service."* See: ASBH 2011: 19–20.

obtaining a second opinion is well known and accepted in other professional practices and generally serves to reinforce, rather than erode, the centrality of the exercise of judgment in the giving of professional advice. This practice remains rare in ethics consultation – nor is it widely discussed in the literature – but where it exists, it should be appropriately regulated as it is in other professional disciplines (for example, by the AMA; see AMA 2016).

Given all of the above, there is no obvious evidence that considerations of Moore's competence, level of expertise or professionalism motivated Finder's intervention in the case at hand or that the scope and limits of his intervention were discussed, understood or agreed to in advance. This I think is highly regrettable when viewed through the lens of professionalization of clinical ethics practice. Few interventions bespeak so forcefully an inherent, if unintended, rejection of professionalism than intrusion into the relationships it exists to serve through the exercise of expert judgment.

The Scope and Limits of Ethics Services

Consider now some of the substantive challenges related to the nature of ethics consultation to which this case also gives rise. Finder, Moore, and the various authors contributing to this book, are all 'ethics' consultants and give ethics advice. This much seems obvious. But the reality on the ground (even among ethicists) is quite different.

Ethics consultants' job is to *"help the consult requester determine if, how and why a certain course of action should or should not be undertaken"* by *"helping the consult requester to identify, analysis and, where appropriate, resolve values uncertainty or conflict"* (ASBH 2011: 3). This is the specific professional service ethics consultants offer. If this is the help that the requester of ethics consultation wants, then a clinical ethics consultation is appropriate. If some other help is sought or is obviously required, then ethics consultation is *not* appropriate. More importantly, that other service should not be rendered by the ethics consultant. In light of these considerations, at least two types of interaction (or more accurately *non*-interaction) engaged in by Finder and Moore require critical comment.

Firstly, not one of the ethics consultation requesters is ever asked by either Moore or Finder how these requesters think ethics consultation might be helpful to them. This is problematic. A major difficulty faced by ethics consultants is a wide-spread lack of knowledge on the part of those who request ethics consultation regarding what it is that ethics consultants actually do. Indeed, there is a lot of positive misunderstanding about the proper scope and limits of the ethics consultants' role and expertise (e.g. the pervasive belief that ethics consultants are or ought to be moral police). Given this fact (or perception), ethics consultants should almost always ask requesters immediately after the facts that form the basis of the consultation request have been narrated," How, as an ethics consultant, might I be helpful to you?" Doing so aims to establish: (a) whether ethics consultation is being appropriately requested and (b) what specific help the requester actually wants. Clarifying requestor expectations at the start of an ethics consultation is vital for avoiding potential misunderstanding on the part of the requester regarding the role of ethics consultation as well as to clarify to the kind of help being sought. It also affords the ethics consultant the opportunity to educate colleagues about the exact nature of the professional expertise ethics consultants have and the services they offer.

In "The Zadeh Scenario," Dr. Broukhim asked Moore for "help" which is rather vaguely characterized as help with talking to the family, providing support to the family, and offering more care for the family. (Finder 2018: 23) At one point, Dr. Broukhim more appropriately characterizes the role of ethics consultation and presumably the 'help' offered as trying to delineate ethical issues in the care of the terminally ill for the family (Finder 2018: 30). Moreover, in the final meeting between Dr. Broukhim, Finder and the family, it is unclear what help Dr. Broukhim wants Finder to provide. Nor is it clear what help Finder intends to provide Dr. Broukhim. In addition, some of the "help" actually provided by Finder and Moore is strikingly inappropriate.

For example, there is Moore's effort to "help" the family by finding a new physician for them when they sacked the neurologist who consulted him. Or again, Moore's actually proposing a clinical plan of care (NG tube placement) as an interim clinical compromise. Finally, Dr. Broukhim's asking Dr. Finder whether providing dialysis would be "reasonable" is another example of a potential confusion on the part of the requester about the role of the ethics consultant and about his own role is an ethical physician. Whether an intervention is 'reasonable' is presumable in the first instance a matter of clinical indication in which regard the physician is the expert, not the ethicist. If the question seeks to address underlying issues related to quality of life, it is not clear that the ethicist has either expertise or authority to give a definitive or even advisory answer.

Interestingly, Dr. Broukhim is aware and informs the family that the reason for ethics involvement is not to "persuade" the family to agree to his preferred treatment plan. He is, of course, right in this respect. And yet it is extremely common for ethics consultants to be consulted to do exactly this, and indeed some of Moore's behaviors toward the family seem designed to do exactly that – and were subsequently perceived by the family to be attempts at persuasion: *"He simply came to get us to say what he wanted to hear"* (Finder 2018: 29). Attempting to persuade patients or families to agree to a particular plan or course of action, presumably because the ethicist has determined that it is the most ethically appropriate course of action in the circumstances is one of the more egregious lapses in professionalism that an ethics consultants may commit. The ability to resist the temptation toward moral partiality (moralism) is perhaps the first and most important endowment of the professional ethics consultants.

Secondly, and most problematically, is the fact that there is little actual "ethics" consultation occurring in this case, i.e., there is little or no attempt made by either Finder or Moore to explicitly identify, analysis or resolve values uncertainty or conflict *qua* its being value uncertainty or conflict. It is one of the primary functions of an ethics consultants to render explicit the ethical or value laden aspects of the uncertainty or conflict which are usually implicit and poorly identified and reflected upon by those who are involved in the case.

In this situation, Dr. Broukhim needs to be specifically asked why he does not want to provide more aggressive treatment to the patient. Does he think it would be ethically wrong to do so? Why does he think it would be ethically wrong? Nothing should be assumed. Ethic consultation should help Dr. Broukhim reflect upon and perhaps develop or mature his own understanding of the goals of his own profession (medicine) and how this does or should influence his own practice of medicine in relation to this particular patient, Mrs. Hamadani. The family needs to know (preferably from Dr. Broukhim himself and not from the ethics consultants) that it is explicitly for ethical reasons (i.e. reason of professional value or core commitment) that he does not want to offer more treatment. The ethics consultant's role consists in facilitating this disclosure in such a way that a practical dilemma is understood in moral terms.

In a similar vein, if the hospital has a futility policy and Dr. Broukhim (or any other physician wants to invoke it), or Finder or Moore recommend that it be invoked, the reasons for the policy's existence, its substantive contents and the conditions for its invocation should have been carefully explained to Mrs. Hamadani's children as an instantiation and application of the institution's values and moral commitments, including a moral commitment to due process. The family too should have been helped to articulate their own values and beliefs and to explain to Dr. Broukhim and his team how those values inform the manner in which they are making decisions for Mrs. Hamadani and their various requests of Dr. Bourkim as her physician.

Each 'side' should have been, in other words, invited to engage the others' concerns precisely as *ethical* concerns, concerns related to core personal and professional values. It is here that an important commonality can be discovered (i.e. a shared commitment to core values) which may enable each side to understand and respect the other better and to move forward, if not *in tandem*, then at least without acrimony and recriminations, each respecting the sincerity with which a position different from their own is held.

For Moore and then Finder, as ethics consultants, not to act intentionally and explicitly in this way is simply to fail to do *ethics* consultation itself. Facilitating moral discourse, specifically understood by participants in the conversation as *moral* discourse, is at the heart of what ethics consultation is about. It is the *telos* of the *praxis*. Ethics consultants exist to help individuals find their moral voice and to listen to the moral voice of others. In and of itself, creating the circumstances for the possibility of authentic moral dialogue represents a singularly successful outcome and is the outcome proper to the consultants' role. Nor is this outcome primarily clinical (i.e. a better choice, because it is a choice of a better medical intervention or better/more reasonable health state). Indeed, in some respects, it is not a clinical outcome at all. It is a moral outcome achieved in and through clinical circumstances. In this regard, professional statements which suggest that the goal of clinical ethics consultation is ultimately improved health care (ASBH 2011: 3) are mistaken.

References

American Medical Association (2016) Code of medical ethics, Current Opinions and Annotations: 2015–2016: opinion 8.041. (Second Opinion)

American Society for Bioethics and Humanities (2011) Core competencies for healthcare ethics consultation, 2nd edn. American Society for Bioethics and Humanities, Glenview

Finder SG (2018) The Zadeh scenario. In: Finder SG, Bliton MJ (eds) Peer review, peer education, and modeling in the practice of clinical ethics consultation: the Zadeh project. Springer, Cham, pp 21–42

Hynds J (2013) The core competences: addressing yesterday's challenges. AJOB 13(2):22–23

Rasmussen LM (2016) Clinical ethicists are not 'ethics' expert-but they do have expertise. J Med Phil 41(4):384–400

This May, or May Not, Be an Ethics Consultation

Tarris Rosell and Britt Johnson

Introduction

We begin with the acknowledgement that with "The Zadeh Scenario," Finder has provided a rich and thick description of what clearly was a challenging opportunity for end-of-life ethics consultation. As such, his narrative now stands as opportunity for us to engage with him in the even more challenging opportunity of post-mortem moral reflection. We have organized our thoughts on this case mostly in the interrogative mode, as questions or queries, and from perspectives informed by our own interests in clinical ethics and healthcare law.

Was This an Ethics Consultation?

Philosophers, especially phenomenologists, do not shy away from the most fundamental questions of any particular occurrence. So we begin by asking: Was this an "ethics consultation," or something else entirely? Perhaps it began as an ethics

T. Rosell (✉)
Center for Practical Bioethics, Department of Bioethics,
Kansas City University of Medicine and Biosciences,
Kansas City, MO, USA

Central Baptist Theological Seminary, Department of History and Philosophy of Medicine,
University of Kansas School of Medicine, Kansas City, KS, USA
e-mail: trosell@practicalbioethics.org

B. Johnson
Department of Bioethics, Kansas City University of Medicine and Biosciences,
Kansas City, MO, USA
e-mail: BJohnson@kcumb.edu

S. G. Finder, M. J. Bliton (eds.), *Peer Review, Peer Education, and Modeling in the Practice of Clinical Ethics Consultation: The Zadeh Project*,
https://doi.org/10.1007/978-3-319-90955-4_7

consultation and became something else, or began as something else and became an ethics consultation. Or maybe it was always something else and only seemed to the "consultant" to be ethics consultation. What was this phenomenon really?

Does an ethics consultation become that on account of someone wearing a name badge that says "Ethics"? Is the essential nature of ethics consultation in the title and role of the ethics consultant? Is human response inextricably linked with or independent of the respondent's title and role? Are there criteria by which we could differentiate an ethics consultation from, say, counseling or emotional care-giving? "The Zadeh Scenario" provides opportunity to ponder such questions, and others.

Perhaps an ethics consultation, as compared to something that is *not* an ethics consultation, is determined mostly by the nature of the request and not so much by that of the response. If so, it is the requestor who ostensibly defines what happens next, whether that be ethics consultation or something else.

Following that thread with particularity to the Zadeh narrative, it is Mr. Zadeh himself, the patient's son, who requests response from a gentleman in the hospital elevator who wears a badge with "Ethics" on it. Three years earlier, Finder's ethics colleague, Dr. Steve Moore, had followed up – and followed up and followed up – on the very first request for ethics consultation in regard to Mrs. Hamadani's situation. Initial consultation request had come from the patient's neurologist, we are told. Subsequent requests came from consulting nephrologists, ICU attending physicians, and social workers. Then the current attending physician, Dr. Broukhim, consults Dr. Moore as well, this request coming just 2 weeks prior to the request from Mr. Zadeh, which marks the beginning of Finder's involvement in the case. Before we turn to Mr. Zadeh, then, the question at hand is, for what were these clinicians looking from someone who wore an "Ethics" badge?

Is Ethics Consultation a Matter of "Stopping"?

The initial requestor had expressed concern to Dr. Moore that this family was inappropriately asking for aggressive intervention of a newly diagnosed cancer. Mrs. Hamadani already suffered from Parkinson's and other diseases, and her cancer had metathesized. Subsequent requestors, we learn, "were concerned that Mrs. Hamadani was suffering, that continued intervention was futile, that her children were making bad decisions" (Finder 2018: 23). Dr. Broukhim, too, asks for Ethics help at the point when he "felt there was nothing more he could do, that Mrs. Hamadani was at the end" (Finder 2018: 23).

It seems that each of these initiators of ethics consultation was looking for help in stopping things they thought ought not to be done to their patient. Or they wanted help to stop family members who were trying to make clinicians do things they believed they ought not to be doing. Is that what ethics consultants do? Stop things from happening?

The language used with patients and families often is that of "stopping" – dialysis, ventilator support, tube-feedings, transfusions, antibiotic therapy, chemotherapy. Otherwise, in ethics we speak of withholding and withdrawing. When clinicians speak of "withdrawing care," we who teach ethics to them are quick to correct their language. It is not *care* that ethically may be withdrawn or stopped, but aggressive treatments that are withdrawn. Stopping ineffective and possibly harmful interventions is one way of caring for patients for whom aggressive palliative care is deemed most appropriate. This is what Mrs. Hamadani's healthcare providers were thinking should be done for her, starting 3 years ago, and yet they seemed unable to accomplish this transition of care due to family opposition to that plan of action. So Ethics is called upon, time and again. Help us stop. Get it to stop. Get them to stop. Isn't this what ethics consultants do, or are supposed to do?

Just as patients have the ethical and legal right to refuse treatment, physicians and healthcare providers are ethically, and sometimes legally, allowed to refuse to treat patients (Timmons 2008). Refusal to treat is limited by law in, for example, the United States' Emergency Medical Treatment and Active Labor Act (Department of Health and Human Services 2001). However, when the patient or patient's surrogate demands treatment that is not medically indicated, a provider need not comply (Timmons 2008). Some laws for individual states within the United States (e.g., Texas) require physicians to transfer the patient's treatment to another provider, while others (e.g., California) allow physicians simply to disregard requests for treatments deemed ineffective (Timmons 2008).

In this case, Dr. Broukhim ethically and legally might refuse to provide some or all treatments requested by Mr. Zadeh and his sisters on behalf of their mother. Her physician would have received a groundswell of collegial support for that course of action, or inaction. There had been a multi-disciplinary chorus of ethics consultation requestors over the years, all looking for things non-beneficial to stop. In lieu of mere refusal, Dr. Broukhim could have sought to transfer Mrs. Hamadani's care to a physician elsewhere with different inclinations as to what might benefit or harm this patient. Alternatively, Dr. Broukhim could have sought legal authority to provide comfort care only. A judge might have been persuaded to assign a guardian ad litem or to designate durable power of attorney to someone other than the patient's son.

However, it is unclear from the narrative that Dr. Broukhim was ready to take such drastic measures. He had a long professional relationship with this patient and family. Like many physicians in that situation, Broukhim was disinclined to cease being Mrs. Hamadani's primary care provider, especially now at the end of life. There is something virtuous about that. How then do things turn out less than good for everyone involved?

For three long years, what providers want stopped keeps going. New aggressive treatments get added rather than all of them being withheld or withdrawn. This occurs despite ethics consultation by Dr. Moore, who also is of a mind to stop aggressive treatment and to enable transition to palliative care. If the initial consultation goal was that of helping everyone stop, it seems to have been unsuccessful. Is that why the patient's son puts in his own subsequent request to Ethics?

Interestingly, Mr. Zadeh's request for ethics consultation, if that's what it was, is also a request to make something stop. But what he asks of Finder is to stop Dr. Moore from engaging in ethics consultation, one that had been happening, on and off, for the past 3 years.

> Your Dr. Moore, he has pestered us, always showing up when my mother has come into the hospital, asking us if we are ready to stop…. And so I beg of you, Doctor, please don't let Dr. Moore see my mother again. My sisters and I do not want him talking with us anymore (Finder 2018: 25–6).

Is Ethics Consultation a Matter of Giving Care?

Mr. Zadeh's request of Finder is not for more ethics consultation, but less – or none at all. How then does this become more of the same? Or did it? Instead of clinical ethics consultation, could Finder's response more accurately be described as a case of non-clinical, non-ethics, emotional care giving?

Perhaps care-giving is what competent and effective ethics consultants actually do. However, caring is not listed as one of the core competencies by the American Society of Bioethics and Humanities in a publication delineating what health care ethics consultants ought to know and do (ASBH 2011: 19–31). Maybe that is an oversight to be corrected. At least in this consultation scenario, Finder demonstrates a competency of care; he writes:

> Several times during these days I stopped by and stuck my head in to say 'Hello' to whoever was there [in the patient's hospital room] …. My aim in doing so was simply to keep tabs, much as Steve had done during prior hospitalizations. But unlike then, and unlike during the earlier part of this hospitalization, I did not inquire about whether they had thought more about CPR and DNAR or if there had been discussions of stopping the dialysis. Rather, I kept my focus on how they were holding up, especially the sisters who also had families for which they had responsibilities. I also asked about their father … (Finder 2018: 36).

Finder is giving care – and also showing compassion, patience, and tolerance, all of which are listed in the ASBH document as essential "traits" for health care ethics consultants (ASBH 2011: 32). He is kind and a good listener, in the normative manner of chaplains and counselors. He seems to care for and about this family.

So this is morality, but is it ethics? Finder is being morally upright, as ethics consultants should be, but is he doing ethics consultation? Was Dr. Moore doing so? What ethics purpose is served by "stopping by" to "keep tabs," without inquiring about stopping treatments deemed futile by clinicians? If the *Core Competencies* of ASBH is considered definitive, care-giving is not really the proper role of one who wears the badge titled, "Ethics." One can exhibit traits of compassion, tolerance, and patience without giving care.

Care-giving also is not what Mr. Zadeh had requested. His request was for ethics consultation to stop, for his family to be left alone, and for the ongoing attention of Dr. Broukhim alone. If the requestor's intent defines the response that is given, then what Finder did, in response, was neither ethics consultation nor emotional care-giving. Yet it seems to us that he did both. Are we mistaken, along with Finder, who clearly presents "The Zadeh Scenario" as a narrative of ethics consultation by one who is at least care-full?

We conclude that a request to stop ethics consultation, when asked of a consultant, does not mean that the response is exactly what the requestor asked for.

Is Ethics Consultation a Matter of Getting Fired?

Dr. Moore's consultation activities did stop when Finder responded. Should that have been the end of this matter, as far as ethics consultation goes? Perhaps. But how would Finder know unless he took things further – stopping by, keeping tabs, asking how things were going for the family? By further response, the consultant learns more about, and then becomes a participant in, a situation of conflict that had gotten Moore and several physicians fired by the family.

The context out of which many ethics consults arise is one of human conflict. Stakeholders are conflicted about means and ends. Not always, but often, these conflicts arise in contexts of end-of-life care, and pertain to starting or stopping aggressive treatment. It was so in the Zadeh narrative. The conflict Mr. Zadeh describes to Finder in their first meeting involved a mistrust and distaste for how Dr. Moore and providers had been treating the patient and her family. Do these clinicians, and this ethics consultant too, not know "what it means to love [a] mother?" (Finder 2018: 25). In particular, Mr. Zadeh wanted Finder to help the family attain some space from what they viewed as overly aggressive and insensitive questioning and badgering by Dr. Moore. Mr. Zadeh was asking for the ability to direct his mother's care as best he could without feeling urged towards options they had previously rejected.

Ethics consultation had been repeatedly requested regarding this patient during previous admissions, and Dr. Moore was the assigned contact for those interactions. Did the family ever ask for any of these consults or request Dr. Moore's presence? Apparently not. Ethically uncomfortable clinicians dial the Ethics pager. It is understandable then that the family views Dr. Moore's mere presence as a harbinger of conflict. Each time they see his face, they expect to be asked to rethink their choices and to cease aggressive treatment. Of course they seek reprieve.

The family's view of Dr. Moore as unwelcome is in line with their general mistrust of hospital staff. None of the children seem to think that their mother would receive the care she needed unless one of them is present at the bedside. The conflictual tension builds with each admission. Some health care providers have refused to participate further in this patient's care.

Finder replaces Moore as the consultant on the case, and attempts to forge a relationship with the family in order to understand their history and current situation. So long as he takes this tack, Finder finds acceptance, or tolerance anyway. Why then does Mr. Zadeh ultimately become as exasperated with Finder as they were with his colleague?

Mr. Zadeh makes clear that his family will make decisions when decisions are needed, i.e., in the crisis moment. Given that at least some of the children are nearly always present with their mother, this may be more reasonable than either ethics consultant and most physicians acknowledged. The narrative gives several indicators of cultural normative difference in regard to making end of life decisions. Majority culture within healthcare has come to value advance care planning, advance directives, and doctors' orders in advance to stop "futile" though default resuscitation attempts. Mr. Zadeh and his sisters reject these tools and processes. Their obstinacy perplexes and perturbs providers, inclusive of those who wear an Ethics badge.

Is the Persian Dr. Broukhim perhaps the only one who truly understands and respects this Persian family's norms for making end of life decisions? Is that why *both* ethics consultants ultimately get fired? This surely is one possible interpretation of Samir Zadeh's final, impassioned and rather angry speech: "Please, Dr. Finder, I do not wish to cause problems, and I apologize for raising my voice. But I do not want to talk about this anymore, and I do not want to talk with anyone else but Dr. Broukhim" (Finder 2018: 41).

If Ethics Consultation Fails, What About the Law?

Patients, and their surrogates, have the ethical and legal right to refuse care from providers. There are few, if any, limitations on this (CSB News 2013). "The patient has the right to make decisions regarding the health care that is recommended by his or her physician. Accordingly, patients may accept or refuse any recommended medical treatment." (AMA 2016) One of the underpinnings of the focus on patient autonomy in the United States is the personal freedoms guaranteed by the nation and states (Beauchamp and Walters 2003: 19). The process of informed consent is built around the pillar of autonomy. Not only are health care providers ethically required to provide complete and accurate information about proposed treatment options, they are to answer the patient's questions, give recommendations, and then provide active support of the patient's decision (Jonsen et al. 2010: 51). To be treated without consent can be a violation of state law; indeed, the most egregious cases of a patient receiving treatment to which she or he has not consented can result in a criminal charge of battery (Trehan and Sankhari 2002).

This situation is more nuanced. The patient's surrogate is not refusing treatment of a particular kind. Rather, Mr. Zadeh asks that certain providers not be involved in his mother's treatment. Just as a patient has no obligation to accept a specific treatment, patients may refuse to be treated by specific providers. When Dr. Moore had stopped by to ask about DNR decisions, the family simply said that it was "not a good time" to talk. When does this polite refusal to chat indicate that the patient or the patient's surrogate has no intention of discussing the matter at all?

The counter-narrative began to take on the persona of someone trying very hard to politely refuse an offer of a date. Not wanting to hurt the other's feelings or to indicate ill will, one might say something like, "Sorry, I'm busy," or simply, "No thanks." But there are times when this indirect refusal is not enough, and the suitor's asking continues. Mannerly rejection might lead to firm insistence with a raised voice – and a perplexed pursuer. So it seems to go for Finder, who is stunned when Mr. Zadeh raises his voice and essentially fires the ethics consultant.

Unfortunately, this is not merely a case of social interaction gone awry. Mr. Zadeh, on behalf of his mother, has the ethical and legal right to refuse "care" from any healthcare provider. Broadly construed, this includes all employees and staff of the medical center, up to and including the ethics consultants. This situation did not reach the level of legal concern; but it leads to yet another ethics question: Ought ethics consultation, like treatment, be undertaken and continued only after documented informed consent by the patient and/or family?

Ethics Consultation as "Paying Attention"

Finder, and several others of us who do clinical ethics consultation, were mentored by philosopher Richard Zaner. Long before an ASBH committee delineated "core competencies" for this practice, Zaner had given us a thick description of the phenomenon referred to as "the clinical encounter." Place a philosopher in that foreign context, and one might further describe "ethics and the clinical encounter," which in 1988 became the title of Zaner's seminal book (Zaner 1988). Using phenomenological method, per the author, the primary activity of hospital foreigners like us is that of paying attention. Indeed, for Zaner and now Finder, too, what is referred to mostly as ethics consultation would be more accurately portrayed as ethics attention. When physicians or social workers or patients or their family call upon us for help, what they are asking us to do, mostly, is to be attentive, to pay attention.

Attentiveness is not our normal way of being in the world, noted Alfred Schutz, one of Zaner's mentors. Mostly we go through life taking things for granted. Citing Schutz, Zaner wrote:

> It has been made wonderfully lucid by Schutz (1973) that the veritable mark of everyday life is what he terms its "taken-for-grantedness." By way of culturally and socially inculcated typifications, we learn in the usual course of affairs simply and habitually to take hosts of things for granted, as going to be more or less as they have proven to be in the past, at least for all practical purposes. Only if something does not conform to our typified expectations are we at all alerted to it specifically, called on to take notice of it, and then to do something about it (Zaner 1988: 66).

So if clinical ethics consultation is fundamentally a practice of paying attention, what specifically does Finder do that constitutes this activity?

His account in "The Zadeh Scenario" indicates that Finder had paid significant attention to this case long before he was asked to get involved directly. Details of this patient's situation had lodged in his memory despite dozens of other cases that must have also begged his time and attention over the course of 3 years. Clearly, there was something about this one that was out of the ordinary, that did not conform to typified expectations of the taken-for-granted world. Hence Dr. Finder pays attention.

When Mr. Zadeh unexpectedly calls his name, Finder understandably pays close attention. "How did this stranger know my name?" Finder wonders. And even when realizing that a name badge has given him away, fulfilling its purpose, the consultant's curiosity has been piqued, memories of this man and his family are elicited, and attention is paid to what happens next.

Certainly there is much evidence of an inordinately attentive ethics consultant in the days and weeks that followed that initial clinical encounter. Finder "stops by" the patient's room time and again, "keeping tabs" on what was happening, asking questions, demonstrating care and compassion by the attention given to strangers.

If Finder's approach to ethics consultation is mostly that of paying attention, there also is evidence in "The Zadeh Scenario" of notable inattention. Surprisingly, lack of attention retrospectively is noted in regard to what for Zaner was the central point of attentive interest in virtually every clinical encounter of which he wrote: the patient. In this narrative, where is the patient?

In Zaner's words: "Careful attention to the complex and subtle ranges of emotive, volitional, and valuational feelings serves to focus a crucial moral question: What is it about any specific patient that evokes, directs, and aims just these specific feelings and serves to orient the discussions, decisions, and actions of others (physicians, family, nurses)?" (Zaner 1988: 56). He might well have added "ethics consultant" to that parenthetical list of "others."

When looking carefully at the contexts out of which clinical ethics consultation arises, for Zaner and others of us, the patient is found at the contextual center. However, Mrs. Hamadani is mostly absent in this consultation activity. There is much interaction with clinicians and family members and the patient's (electronic and paper) chart. There is little if any mention of interacting with the patient herself, not even during the time immediately following dialysis when "her mental status did improve somewhat, and there were points when she was purposeful" (Finder 2018: 35). Assumedly, she still was not communicative; but what attempts by the consultant were made to communicate with her, to observe and reflect on the patient herself – and not just those who speak for her? How did the patient look? What was she doing? Did she appear comfortable or in pain? Was she awake, seeing, hearing, or responding in any way?

Conclusion

After reading "The Zadeh Scenario," Finder the ethics consultant's lengthy and fascinating narrative, we feel that we know the three Zadeh children, can picture them. But there is no picture or sense of their mother, even though she is the patient. Why not? Why do we not even think to raise the question until this late in a retrospective reflection on "The Zadeh Scenario"? It seems that none of us have been sufficiently attentive to the patient. Perhaps she had been too much "taken for granted"? If so, this is an unexpected and atypical lapse on the part of Finder, whose thick description narrative otherwise takes very little for granted.

Albert Jonsen has written that ethics consultation involves "thoughtful, compassionate, honest attention ... given to a deeply troubling, perplexing human problem" (Ford and Dudzinski 2008: xix). By that definition, what Finder documents as his primary activity – indeed, this entire retrospective venture to which others of us have been invited – is the epitome of ethics consultation. It is, in fact, the act of paying attention.

As such, there is no tidy ending point for something that was begun as a request for help in stopping something or someone. Note the irony of this. As long as attention is paid, there is no stopping whatsoever, and the ethics consultation goes on and on. By Jonsen's definition, even the writing of this chapter is a sort of ethics consultation in the context of an unfinished narrative.

References

American Medical Association (2016) Code of medical ethics, Current Opinions and Annotations: 2015–2016: opinion 10.01

American Society for Bioethics and Humanities (2011) Core competencies for healthcare ethics consultation, 2nd edn. American Society for Bioethics and Humanities, Glenview

Beauchamp TL, Walters L (eds) (2003) Contemporary issues in bioethics, 6th edn. Thomson/Wadsworth, Belmont

CBS News (2013) Patients refusing care from nurses of different race one of medicine's "Open Secret." Available at: http://www.cbsnews.com/news/patients-refusing-care-from-nurses-of-different-race-one-of-medicines-open-secrets/

Department of Health and Human Services, Office of Inspector General (2001) The Emergency Medical Treatment and Labor Act. The enforcement process (Pub. no. OEI-09-98-00221). Available at http://oig.hhs.gov/oei/summaries/b510.pdf. Accessed July 2001

Finder SG (2018) The Zadeh scenario. In: Finder SG, Bliton MJ (eds) Peer review, peer education, and modeling in the practice of clinical ethics consultation: the Zadeh project. Springer, Cham, pp 21–42

Ford P, Dudzinski D (eds) (2008) Complex ethics consultations: cases that haunt us. Cambridge University Press, New York

Jonsen AR, Siegler M, Winslade WJ (2010) Clinical ethics: a practical approach to ethical decisions in clinical medicine, 7th edn. McGraw Hill, New York

Timmons D (2008) Medical futility: can a physician unilaterally terminate treatment for a patient when he believes further measures to be futile? Law Library Student-Authored Works, Georgia State College of Law. Paper 66

Trehan SP, Sankhari D (2002) Medical professional, patient and the law: the institute of law and ethics in medicine, 2nd edn. National Law School of India University, Bangalore, pp 57–68

Zaner RM (1988) Ethics and the clinical encounter. Prentice Hall, Englewood Cliffs

PART THREE REFLECTIONS ON METHOD IN RESPONSE TO THE ZADEH SCENARIO AND PART TWO

Brief Summary of the Essays in Part Three

The authors of Part Three were invited to reflect on and respond to the set of interactions, issues, and criticisms addressed by the authors of Part Two and to identify the relevant features, the appraisals, and assessment of the methods that emerge among the Scenario and that first set of responses. It is important to note that we deliberately and insistently encouraged the authors of Part Three to critically examine several questions, especially in regard to the ways that methods of inquiry used in the practice of ethics consultation might allow for a careful appraisal of cultural, social, political, institutional, and moral attitudes – embedded as they are in clinical routines and practices. We posed that set of questions because those attitudes not only shape the ways that circumstances are then considered to pose "ethical problems" but they contribute to both the variety of languages and to the different ways that moral and ethical matters are framed and understood (that is, taken for granted) in those different contexts. This point can be readily appreciated by simply noticing that requests for clinical ethics consultation, while coming from many different clinical situations, are constructed around what are already perceived as moral or ethical problems, but as these are frequently not well articulated, they are more akin to moral experiences, feelings, even beliefs evoked in specific situations (DuVal et al. 2004; Wasson et al. 2016).

In her essay, "Not Principlism nor Casuistry, Not Narrative Ethics nor Clinical Pragmatism: A Case for Proceduralism," Courtenay Bruce provides a clear example of identifying themes across the variations among the essays in the preceding section. She then suggests that there is "a common thread in all of the peer reviewers' assessments ('proceduralism')" (Bruce 2018: 114) [citation] through her review and comparison of principlism, casuistry, narrative, and clinical pragmatism. She also critically examines Tarzian's essay to propose a kind of proceduralism that "allows for internal consistency and justificatory force to the extent that certain steps should be followed and justifications provided if these steps are not followed" (Bruce 2018: 123). Bruce goes on to offer several elements that must be explicitly integrated into the processes of clinical ethics consultation. The consultant should "identify the nature of the ethical concern early, including how one, as the clinical ethicist, could or should assist in this case" (Bruce 2018: 124). Likewise, Bruce says, "to move a case toward resolution, it is important to identify which interventions or actions are considered inappropriate and for what reasons" (Bruce 2018: 124). Bruce also provides a particularly interesting requirement that the consultant needs to be explicit about the actual approach utilized, and if the consultant does not follow one or another of the steps in that process, then justification for not doing so should be provided.

Next, Mark Aulisio raises for consideration the "(Meta-) Methodological Lessons for Ethics Consultation." While sharing the explicit concern to address elements of methods that might be compatible with a wide variety of specific standpoints and approaches, Aulisio raises another challenge in order to highlight the need to address what he refers to as "normative dimensions" of decision-making authority, including a focus on care also linked to standards of care, familial relationships, and patient autonomy. In keeping with Zaner's idea that an ethicist is an "interpreter of texts," Aulisio pays close attention to the Scenario and then suggests several ways to engage the matter of differences. For instance, he says that one of the differences was "less over the value of respecting and caring for one's parents and more over what it means to respect and care for one's parents" (Aulisio 2018: 129). From there, however, Aulisio does not interpret those differences in "what it means" so much as he begins to translate. This shift occurs as he translates the appraisal of meanings into rules or maxims for guidelines, thus indicating a more extensive scope for his considerations about methodology for using or applying such guidelines.

George Agich, in his chapter, "Narrative and Method in Ethics Consultation," begins by describing a series of key elements of what method "is" in the actual "doing" of ethics consultation, such that method serves as the lens through which to view the field of clinical ethics. For Agich, what cannot be ignored or obscured is the central relevance of rules located by and enacted in ethics consultation practice. Because rules "are dependent upon that practice for their ultimate meaning and justification," Agich goes on to say that "as a practice ethics consultation essentially is nothing more than the various actions that constitute the meanings of the individuals involved in performing the ethics consultation" (Agich 2018: 143). Agich shows that "the meaningfulness of statements made in the course of ethics consultation are therefore fundamentally dependent upon the wider set of social meanings that provide a framework of acceptance of the particular doings of ethics consultants by patients, families, and health professionals" (Agich 2018: 143). Agich also highlights a concern that although "ethics consultation services have become accepted in healthcare institutions, the consultations in many places take on a ceremonial aspect," which can distort and obscure other significant forms of meaning (Agich 2018: 143). Accordingly, for Agich, the sociality of actual clinical engagement is key for engaging in any legitimate sense of evaluation of clinical ethics practice. Agich then goes on to cogently and briefly outline several key elements that are directly relevant to and deserve inclusion in any adequate assessment of peer review.

In the final chapter of Part Three, "Standardizing the Case Narrative," Lisa Rasmussen delves more critically into the very notion of narrative composition and the ways that various formats of presenting clinical ethics practice already shape what is seen as relevant for any evaluation of such practice. She then identifies one central issue at the core of the Zadeh Project. Rasmussen notes, sharply, "if all we have to evaluate the case is a written report, and we lack a standard for evaluating the written report, we lack a true standard for evaluating a case. And so, questions about method in consultation become, under an attestation model, questions about method in consultation summaries. We must articulate the links between what should be done in a consultation and what must be included in a case report" (Rasmussen 2018: 153). To illustrate her point, she focuses explicitly on the range of observations for two categories found in Part Two – concerns about proceduralism as articulated by Frolic and Rubin, Armstrong, Tarzian, and Hynds, and considerations associated with feminism and multicultural concerns which are taken up by Armstrong, Tarzian, and Rosell and Johnson. The implication is that similar linkages must be identified and established among normative positions in the multiple arenas of ethics consultation in health care in order to understand the extremely divergent array of actual responsibilities that could be constructed.

References

DuVal G, Clarridge B, Gensler G, Danis M (2004) A national survey of U.S. Internists' experience with ethical dilemmas and ethics consultation. J Gen Intern Med 19(3):251–258

Wasson K, Anderson E, Hagstrom E et al (2016) What ethical issues really arise in practice at an academic medical center? A quantitative and qualitative analysis of clinical ethics consultations from 2008 to 2013. HEC Forum 28(3):217–228

Not Principlism nor Casuistry, Not Narrative Ethics nor Clinical Pragmatism: A Case for Proceduralism

Courtenay R. Bruce

Neither the method employed by philosophy nor theology nor anthropology nor history nor law nor any other methods that contribute to scholarship in medical ethics describe the blackbird called medical ethics in its entirety. But by examining a moral question from the vantage point of several different methods, one gains a richer understanding of that moral question, and a better grasp of an answer.

—*Sugarman and Sulmasy, Methods in Medical Ethics, p. 4*

Introduction

Finder allows the story arc of his case to intricately and poetically unfold, moving across various interpersonal domains and temporal sequences. Contrary to most case descriptions wherein the narrator and reader are detached, in "The Zadeh Scenario" Finder situates the case fully within the interpersonal context in which clinical ethicists operate, providing important contextual elements related to: dialogue, environment, emotionality, nonverbal and verbal cues, and stakeholders' perspectives. Without this degree of detail, the peer reviewers of Part Two would not have been able to analyze what occurred during the case and what could (or should) have been done differently. The reviewers were afforded an opportunity to critically appraise and reflect on the clinical ethicist's actions because of Finder's level of detail.

One of the most striking features of the reviewers' commentaries is that their assessments are largely devoid of ethical nomenclature like consequences, rights, and virtues. Their focus is practical and process-oriented rather than theory-driven. They, like Finder, often do not discuss the "ethics" of the case in any traditional

C. R. Bruce (✉)
Institute of Academic Medicine, Houston Methodist Hospital, Houston, TX, USA

Texas A&M University College of Medicine, Houston, TX, USA
e-mail: crbruce@houstonmethodist.org

S. G. Finder, M. J. Bliton (eds.), *Peer Review, Peer Education, and Modeling in the Practice of Clinical Ethics Consultation: The Zadeh Project*,
https://doi.org/10.1007/978-3-319-90955-4_8

sense, but spend considerable effort expounding on the lives, sufferings, stories, and doubts (personal and professional) that permeate the case. This focus does not imply that the reviewers lack a method; rather, their analyses suggest that their methods are interpersonal in nature, ones involving an interpretative process or a deliberate uncovering of ethical meanings (Agich 2005). A common feature that undergirds all of their assessments seems to be an implicit belief that engaging in patient care entails finding a clinically-feasible (but process-driven) solution.

In what follows, I will first outline what many considered the four most prominent (at least in the clinical ethics literature) methods for "doing" clinical ethics. For each I will also consider if, and how, the method may have been utilized in the peer reviews of Part Two. Where reviewers employ different methods within their analyses, or where they are unclear in their methods, I will draw attention to it. I will then shift attention to the method that I perceive as a common thread in all of the peer reviewers' assessments ("proceduralism"). This common thread can be seen as a combination of two existing methods, or even as an entirely new method. This new method, as I will explain, seems to be utilized in order to seek deeper understanding of the relationships between the experiences of individuals and their social frameworks, much like the narrative method. However, this method goes beyond the traditional story-focus of a narrative method by identifying and anchoring the problem within an ethical framework in which the clinical ethicist has an explicit goal of formulating and achieving an acceptable solution by using discrete process-steps. This method thus seeks to overcome some of the indeterminacy and tentativeness of stories by incorporating a procedural, objective layer within the ethical framework.

Traditional Clinical Ethics Methods

"Method" here refers to a systematic procedure, technique, or mode of inquiry employed during the clinical ethics consultation (Sugarman and Sulmasy 2001: 5). There is considerable debate within the clinical ethics community about *the* method for conducting ethics consultation, with four main contenders likely being principlism, casuistry, narrative ethics, and clinical pragmatism (Kuczewski 1998). Each of the methods vary in their theoretical grounding, in their process, and in their practical implications (Hurst et al. 2006).

Principlism

Originating in the late 1970s and early 1980s, the principlist approach to ethical decision-making has dominated Western bioethics for many years. The approach manifested through several publications around that time, including the *Belmont*

Report, which identified basic principles that should guide research involving human subjects. Several books defended a principlist framework, most notably the work of Beauchamp and Childress (1979).

Central Tenets

(1) Ethical principles (e.g., autonomy, nonmaleficence, beneficence, and justice) and their guiding rules are central to ethical decision-making; (2) A decision is morally justifiable if that decision is consistent with the principles and their theoretical underpinnings; (3) The justificatory force of a decision can be measured by the degree to which it achieves an overall cohesion of all of the elements of the decision-making process (McCarthy 2003).

Explanation

The principlist approach holds that ethical theories (such as utilitarianism and deontology) are too general to guide specific actions, especially as they relate to clinical ethics consultation. Theories, however, give rise to more specific principles, and these principles are *prima facie* duties or obligations that the moral agent should perform. When duties conflict, like in a case where a patient with decision-making capacity requests treatment that is not considered medically beneficial (a conflict between autonomy and beneficence, at least at face value), we may not be able to fulfill all of our obligations. A conflict between duties requires us to balance the conflicting principles and determine which one has more weight. No single principle, duty, or rule has *a priori* priority (Kuczewski 1998). This weighing and balancing is referred to as "reflective equilibrium" (Beauchamp and Childress 1979). When choosing a solution, the infringement upon any one principle or duty must be minimized as much as possible, and we should seek to minimize the negative effects of the infringement.

Strengths and Limitations

This method for ethical decision-making uses an objective approach, allowing for replicability and transparent processes. The approach is versatile. Specifically, by describing the obligations as "*prima facie*," the principles can be considered morally equivalent at face value but can be given priority in certain situations (McCarthy 2003). Criticisms about this method generally center on its application. Some have argued that the method is too theoretical and cannot be easily applied to clinical realities in any sort of practical way: "ethical principles offer limited guidance for the clinical tasks of caring for patients" (Block and Billings 1994).

Commentaries' Appeals to Principlism

Principlism is rarely discussed in most of the reviewers' assessments, which could suggest that this ethical framework is outdated, has limited applicability in their analyses, or that they found other methods more useful when analyzing the case. Most likely, their lack of discussion about principlism reflects a combination of these and other factors. Where principlism is invoked, it is implicit in discussion about ethically appropriate treatments. For instance, Tarzian writes: "The difficulty in identifying which 'grey zone' interventions qualify as 'medically inadvisable' rests on judgments about which goals for Mrs. Hamadani are of 'controversial value'" (Tarzian 2018: 81). Tarzian appeals to beneficence-based judgments by calling for a clinical evaluation of the interventions that would be empirically, quantifiably medically beneficial to achieve physiologic and ethical goals. Further, Hynds writes, "most problematically [in Finder's report]…is that there is little actual 'ethics' consultation occurring in this case…no attempt...to identify, analyze, or resolve values uncertainty or conflict *qua* its being value uncertainty or conflict….The family needs to know...that it is explicitly for ethical reasons (i.e. reason of professional value or core commitment) that [Dr. Broukhim] does not want to offer more treatment" (Hynds 2018: 95–6). In essence, Hynds is looking for consultative method, some framework by which to analyze the case and reach a judgment, and he appeals to the virtue of professional integrity in doing so. Likewise, all of the commentaries mention the importance of hearing the patient's voice for autonomy-enhancing purposes, which is consistent with principlism.

Casuistry

Casuistry became popular in the 1990s as an alternative to theory-driven application of principles by viewing clinical ethics as dealing with concrete problems and unique cases (Agich 2005). Unlike principlism, casuists do not apply principles to cases in an inferential manner. Jonsen (who may be said to be the individual most responsible for re-introducing casuistry to the bioethics community) defines casuistry as:

> The interpretation of moral issues, using procedures of reasoning based on paradigms and analogies, leading to the formulation of expert opinion about the existence and stringency of particular moral obligations, framed in terms of rules or maxims that are general but not universal or invariable, since they hold good with certainty only in the typical conditions of the agent and circumstance of action. (Jonsen 1991a, b: 297)

Central Tenets

Jonsen identifies three stages of moral reasoning in using casuistry: (1) Identify the case and its relevant features, including the moral problems; (2) Compare the case to other cases, especially paradigmatic cases; (3) Use analogies to determine the fit between the case at hand and the paradigm cases (Kuczewski 1998; Jonsen 1995).

Explanation

Casuistry differs from principlism in that no single principle, rule of thumb, or maxim can be affirmed. Casuistry holds that principles are too vague. The ethicist discovers and elucidates principles by exploring cases. That is, principles cannot guide action until content is provided through paradigmatic cases (Kuczewski 1998). The clinical ethicist should consider cases where the principle applies and contrast them with cases where the principle could be suspended.

Strengths and Limitations

Casuistry is persuasive in its practicality, especially given its emphasis on actual clinical ethics cases. It also has the benefit of working with principlism, and most advocates of casuistry do not view the methods as mutually exclusive or incongruent. That is, many advocates of casuistry view case methods as more basic and more reliable than maxims or principles, with rules coming into play in order to give direction once the case is evaluated and compared. On this point, Jonsen uses an example where he analogizes a bicycle to a practical judgment and a hot-air balloon to ethical theory: "The balloon of theory can give us orientation of mind and exhilaration of moral imagination. However, we are not tethered to the balloon; we do not need it for moment-to-moment directions through ethical problems. The balloon is an occasional extravagance. The bicycle is daily transportation and exercise" (Jonsen 1991a, b: 16). The criticisms surrounding casuistry include questions of bias and the constitution of paradigmatic cases. Bias can arise in casuistry when: describing the selection criteria for a certain case, stating the problem to be examined and exemplified, choosing a comparison case, and identifying the selected paradigmatic case (Kopelman 1994).

Commentaries' Appeals to Casuistry

While there is no systematic appeal to casuistry within the commentaries, there are several times when commenters seem to make some sort of casuistic-like appeals. What remains unclear, however, is why a particular perspective is presented as paradigmatic, and why the specific features are identified as *ethically* relevant. To the extent that casuistry is employed, it is generally invoked in a very legalistic sense. For example, Rosell and Johnson write: "Just as patients have the ethical and legal right to refuse treatment, physicians and healthcare providers are ethically, and sometimes legally, allowed to refuse to treat patients... Some laws for individual states within the United States (e.g. Texas) require physicians to transfer the patient's treatment to another provider...In this case..." (Rosell and Johnson 2018: 101). They thus seem to be using legal statutes as paradigms with which to examine the scenario Finder presents, but it is unclear how these statutes would be applied in this situation – let alone whether these laws actually *are* applicable in this case. What is needed to answer that question is more detail relating to how or why such laws should be applied.

Narrative Ethics

Narrative ethics deploys narratives and methods derived from world literature as a basis for assessment. Narrative ethics calls for masterful skills in observation, interpretation, and elucidation of patients' values and experiences (Hunter et al. 1995).

Central Tenets

The study of narrative ethics is young, making it difficult to discern a clear articulation of its central tenets. McCarthy provides perhaps the clearest and most concise version: "(1) Every moral situation is unique and unrepeatable and its meaning cannot be fully captured by appealing to law-like universal principles; (2) Any decision…is justified in terms of its fit with the individual life story or stories of the patient; (3) The objective of the task of justification in 2 is not necessarily to unify moral beliefs and commitment, but to open up dialogue…[and] explore tensions" (McCarthy 2003: 67).

Explanation

An essential premise behind the narrative approach is a belief that the patient's story (or narrative) is a rich source of qualitative data that could be used to inform the clinical ethicist's assessment and analysis. In most ethics consultations, elucidating a patient's moral life story is a key procedural task for the clinical ethicist. Indeed, the moral values and life circumstances of patients will often need to be elucidated and carefully documented as part of the information-gathering efforts that occur early on during the ethics consultation. As Dubler and colleagues describe:

> The medical team is the expert on illness and disease, but the family is the expert on 'Mama.' Plumbing their perceptions and encouraging them to tell their stories helps to bring the patient to the center of the discussion and gives voice to and empowers the family amidst the alien discourse of medicine. (Dubler et al. 2009: 26)

To elucidate the patient's story, the ethicist uses open-ended elucidation questions. The most credible stories are those that adequately and fully capture significant events in a person's life (McCarthy 2003; Brody and Clark 2014). Narrativists do not focus on trying to reduce competing perspectives or to reconcile them; rather, they focus more on bringing as many people into the dialogue as possible to optimize chances of respecting all the persons involved in the case. Empathetic listening and support are considered paramount in this process (McCarthy 2003).

Strengths and Limitations

Narrative ethics poses a nice contrast with principlism. The narrative approach seeks to incorporate multiple perspectives, which is important for inclusion purposes and for conducting a robust analysis. Narrative ethics also introduces the idea that ethics should not be only concerned with reducing discord. But this "strength" also serves as a point of criticism. Specifically, there is an element of indeterminacy in stories and those who are interested in narrative ethics are most interested in enduring moral character and less interested in what a person should do (Brody and Clark 2014). The challenge in clinical ethics, however, is that indeterminacy is typically unsatisfactory for the consult requestor. He or she *needs* to know what to do, otherwise a consult request would never have been placed. Indeterminacy drove the consult request, and the case should not be "resolved" by simply introducing more uncertainty.

Commentaries' Appeals to Narrative

Finder's account in "The Zadeh Scenario" and the peer reviewers' responses are replete with narrative examples, with each one of them embracing some form of narrative. Indeed, Finder's conclusion echoes narrativist sentiments: "We often proceed as if endings need to be smooth and unitary, all the loose strings tied up together into an easily digestible resolution. But why should that be when the very context, and content, of such meetings concern a kind of coming apart, a dissolution, an undoing of a moment that has lasted possibly 83 years?" (Finder 2018: 42). We also see that references to "the narrative" or "story" appear at least ten different times among all of the commenters' assessments, with each commentary mentioning it at least once. For instance, Armstrong writes: "Finder's polished skills of careful attention and mindful appreciation in recounting the 'doing' of an ethics consult thus provide something of an anthropological account—telling us who went where and the content of several weighty conversations" (Armstrong 2018: 63). And Frolic & Rubin write that "[Finder] offers us a case narrative into which he has chosen to place himself squarely and explicitly…individuals inevitably become 'characters' based on how other people perceive them and the social roles they play" (Frolic and Rubin 2018: 47).

On the one hand, the reviewers' applaud Finder for the richness in which he tells the story. They also credit him for using open and well-crafted questions that allows him to elucidate the family's story. This prompting, in turn, allows him to more fully understand the family's moral perspectives. On the other hand, however, they are quick to identify one story that is notably lacking in the case presentation: that of the patient. Rosell & Johnson write, "there also is evidence in 'The Zadeh Scenario' of notable inattention…In this narrative, where is the patient?" (Rosell and Johnson 2018: 106). Armstrong writes: "It is concerning that "The Zadeh Scenario" narrative fails to explicitly identify and analyze whose wishes are being expressed, instead focusing on the role of the patient's children in decision-making" (Armstrong 2018: 68).

Clinical Pragmatism

A fourth model of ethics consultation adopts a process model of moral problem-solving and deliberation. Here, the facts of the case unfold and are assessed in a dynamic process of inquiry in order to achieve a resolution that is within the range of an ethically appropriate plan of care. It is considered dynamic in the sense that it concerns interactions between clinicians, patients or their surrogates, and the clinical ethicist.

Central Tenets

This model uses a systematic approach involving the following steps: (1) Assess the patient's situation (capacity, values, beliefs, preferences, and prognosis) and determine the point of ethical concern; (2) Determine the appropriate goals of medical care, including what types of treatment are appropriate or inappropriate and on what basis. (3) Arrive at a clinically and ethically appropriate plan (Jonsen et al. 2006; Miller et al. 1996; Dewey 1944).

Explanation

Borrowed heavily from Dewey's work, clinical pragmatics treats ethical theories (consequentialism, deontology, and virtues) as tools to guide problem-solving. The emphasis is on reconstructing ethical thinking to integrate it with clinical judgment. By focusing on concrete problems and practical considerations to facilitate resolution of the case, it retains clinical significance. In other words, this approach adopts a process model to solve moral problems, instead of a "judgment" model that is typical of casuistry and principlism (Miller et al. 1996).

Strengths and Limitations

The most salient positive feature of this model is that it attends to the interpersonal nature of ethics consultation, while also recognizing that there are substantive decisions to make. In this way, it goes beyond narrative ethics by focusing on actually resolving the case at hand. Further, by merging ethical and clinical thinking, it is achieves goals of ethicists and clinicians alike (Miller et al. 1996). A drawback of this model is that it does little to specify the actual steps that should be taken other than broad-level enumeration. It emphasizes the importance of interpersonal relations, but stops short of discussing how stories should be integrated within the decision-making calculus, or how conflict-resolution skills or ethical appeals should be applied.

Commentaries' Appeals to Clinical Pragmatism

The clearest examples of this approach can be gleaned from Tarzian's commentary. The word "process" appears as the third word in her assessment, setting the stage for what is to come. She identifies several process measures she would have implemented in an ethics consultation that appear not to have been implemented by Finder. Like several of her peer reviewers' commentaries, she emphasizes the importance of identifying with what a requestor wants help and then clarifying how the ethics consultant could or could not assist. She, like others, believes this was not done in Finder's case or, at the very least, was not clearly articulated in "The Zadeh Scenario." She goes on to write,

> From this point on, however, there is ambiguity in several procedural aspects of how this consultation was handled. First, it was not entirely clear how limits on Dr. Moore's involvement would be communicated to other staff... Second, it's not clear that Finder has clarified what role he will play in the case. (Tarzian 2018: 79)

In short, Tarzian seems implicitly to believe that, because certain process standards were neither acknowledged nor adhered to, it is unclear whether the case was fully resolved, how the ethics consultant contributed to the case, and whether the healthcare professionals involved in this case felt supported by Finder's involvement.

Reflecting a New Method: Learning from the Peer Reviews

While the clinical ethics literature is filled with appeals to, or arguments for or against, the above briefly discussed methods, in their responses to "The Zadeh Scenario," the reviewers consistently appeal to both procedural standards and narrative themes throughout. This combination of pragmatic and narrative appeals serves a crucial role: it makes up for the shortcomings of each of the methods. Whether intentional or not, the method suggested by these peer reviews is persuasive in its idiosyncrasies because it draws on the best features of each respective method and avoids the weaknesses.

Consider Tarzian's peer review. She is explicit about commitment to pragmatism when she writes, "Attending mindfully to the process of how health care ethics consultation is done is just as important as demonstrating that ethics consultants have requisite skills and knowledge" (Tarzian 2018: 75). And yet, at the same time,

Tarzian seems to be quite cognizant of the fact that this approach is too linear, too non-descript. Its emphasis on practical considerations does little to explicate the process steps to be taken or avoided. Hence, Tarzian, goes beyond pragmatism by also appealing to professional standards (articulated by ASBH and PHEEP) as her structural basis. She then lists defined procedural elements, as enumerated by these professional organizations, with one step including narrative interpretation. Here are the procedural elements she describes:

1. **Clarify the consult request**. Why is the requestor requesting an ethics consultation? What is it he or she perceives as the point of ethical concern? What degree of involvement is he or expecting? (This point was reiterated by several reviewers, suggesting they consider it to be a critical preliminary process-step.)
2. **Communicate how colleagues' roles might be limited**. What might clinicians expect of colleagues? How will they be interacting with the ethics consultant? Who will "stay on" the case, and in what capacity?
3. **Determine what role should be taken during a family meeting**. Will the clinical ethicist lead the family meeting? Facilitate conversation? Observe the meeting? On what basis is this judgment to be made, and to whom should this be communicated?
4. **If the point of concern is one involving medically inappropriate treatments, then clarify which treatments are considered inappropriate and on what basis this judgment is made**. What is the desired goal of the intervention? Can it be achieved? Is there agreement among the clinicians about the appropriateness or inappropriateness of a treatment?
5. **Particularly in cases where there are numerous healthcare professionals involved, and where there is a high degree of intellectual or emotional weariness, consider a team only meeting to** (a) identify which treatments are inappropriate and on what basis; (b) streamline and facilitate communication; (c) delineate options; and (d) formulate a plan of care that is shared and agreed-upon.
6. **Appeal to professional standards, literature, law, and professional guidance statements to guide clinical ethicists' consultative activities and provide justifications for actions taken.** (This approach runs along similar lines as casuistry.)
7. **It is important to unpack clinicians, patients, and surrogates' perspectives, thoughts, and beliefs (appealing to narrative ethics**). The narrative approach comes up less in Tarzian's review than it does in the other commentaries, but there are elements of it throughout her commentary: (a) "While Dr. Finder recognizes these cultural differences in his write-up of "The Zadeh Scenario," it's unclear whether or how he addressed these conflicts in his role as the ethics consultant" (Tarzian 2018: 80); (b) "Perhaps like the Iranian physician…Dr. Broukhim struggles with what *T'aarof* demands in these situations" (Tarzian 2018: 82); (c) "He also would not be the first oncologist who needs support accepting his own patient's death and guidance in how to help families do the same" (Tarzian 2018: 83);

8. **There needs to be an attempt to resolve the case, move it along, and address the underlying ethical issues.** As Tarzian states: "Being a good listener is necessary—but not sufficient—for being an effective ethics consultant" (Tarzian 2018: 83). More than just listening to stories, ethics consultants must actually use those stories within a procedural framework to address value-laden uncertainty or ethical conflict. The narrative component, then, is just a layer, a step, within the procedural framework required for conducting an ethics consultation.
9. **To address the issue, the ethics consultant may need to use a combination of active listening skills and conflict-resolution skills.** The conflict resolution skills may take a form of mediation (perhaps entailing a compromise where it is ethically permissible) or a more directive communication approach (like defining boundaries on what constitutes appropriate/inappropriate medical treatment and what therapies will or will not be offered). This also could be conceptualized as extending beyond simple narrative ethics by boundary-drawing, where appropriate.

Indeed, each peer reviewer in Part Two invokes narrative and procedural components. Each uses at least some professional standards to serve as the basis for the inclusion of procedural elements. So what is this method? Is it simply a combination of narrative ethics and pragmatism? I suggest it is a far more particularized, systematic approach than either one of those methods call for. It is pragmatic, but is more than just practical. It is less about just, so to speak, "being in the trenches" by interacting with clinicians and patients/surrogates, which is precisely what the pragmatic approach calls for, and instead calls for being in the trenches in a very systematic, procedural-oriented way that is in keeping with agreed-upon professional standards (to the extent there are agreed-upon professional standards, articulated by ASBH). Additionally, it is less about just hearing the stories, which is precisely what the narrative method calls for, and instead relies on stories to formulate the basis for clinical ethicists' recommendations and action-oriented "plans" or "steps" for resolving the case. Narrative ethics is not used as a singular consultation methodology; rather, it is used as one procedural step among many that need to be taken to conduct the consult well.

In short, this method, which may more properly be referred to as "proceduralism," is distinct from both narrative ethics and clinical pragmatism. Proceduralism allows for internal consistency and justificatory force to the extent that certain steps should be followed and justifications provided if these steps are not followed. It is based on professional standards but allows for exceptions that are case-specific. One could theorize that a shift towards proceduralism occurs because of (or ancillary to) professionalization movements of clinical ethics. The creation and promulgation of a standard process for certifying clinical ethicists leads to a desire for a structural, procedural framework to guide clinical ethicists' methods. Furthermore, such an approach is conductive to checkboxes and criteria, performance improvement, and overall quality improvement efforts that serve as the hallmark of contemporary healthcare.

Conclusion

The reviewers in Part Two employ bits and pieces of several different methods, drawing on those features they find helpful, while avoiding those features that prove to be less helpful in their analyses. They apply very little principlism (only implicitly, really) and casuistry. Where they use casuistry, it is often appealed to somewhat incompletely or irreverently. In contrast, their reviews contain several narrative and pragmatic elements, which I suggest might be indicative of a shift towards a new method, one that echoes narrative and pragmatism approaches while using procedural standards to orient their method.

More work is needed to confirm whether this is an entirely new method or whether it is simply a combination of narrative ethics and pragmatism. In the interim, I can make some preliminary recommendations for peer review of clinical ethics consultations, based on what I am able to extrapolate from my colleagues' reviews. First, it is important to be deliberate and explicit in the approach taken. If one of the procedural steps enumerated above is not taken, then the consultant should provide a justification for doing so. Second, identify the nature of the ethical concern early, including how one, as the clinical ethicist, could or should assist in this case. Third, be explicit in one's role by explaining what one will be doing in the case and why. Fourth, in order to move a case toward resolution, it is important to identify which interventions or actions are considered inappropriate and for what reasons. In the absence of these and other activities enumerated more fully above, it may be difficult fully to evaluate the work of clinical ethics colleagues, other than to say there is always value in listening to patients, surrogates, and clinicians.

References

Agich GJ (2005) What kind of doing is clinical ethics? Theor Med Bioeth 26(1):7–24

Armstrong K (2018) Telling about engagement is not enough: seeking the "ethics" of ethics consultation in clinical ethics case reports. In: Finder SG, Bliton MJ (eds) Peer review, peer education, and modeling in the practice of clinical ethics consultation: the Zadeh project. Springer, Cham, pp 63–73

Beauchamp JF, Childress TL (1979) Principles of biomedical ethics. Oxford University Press, New York

Block SD, Billings JA (1994) Patient requests to hasten death. Evaluation and management in terminal care. Arch Intern Med 154(18):2039–2047

Brody H, Clark M (2014) Narrative ethics: a narrative. Hast Cent Rep 44(1 Suppl): S7–S11

Dewey J (1944) Human nature and conduct. Published for the United States Armed Forces Institute by Henry Holt, New York

Dubler NN, Webber MP, Swiderski DM et al (2009) Charting the future. Credentialing, privileging, quality, and evaluation in clinical ethics consultation. Hastings Cent Rep 39(6):23–33

Finder SG (2018) The Zadeh scenario. In: Finder SG, Bliton MJ (eds) Peer review, peer education, and modeling in the practice of clinical ethics consultation: the Zadeh project. Springer, Cham, pp 21–42

Frolic A, Rubin SB (2018) Critical self-reflection as moral practice: a collaborative meditation on peer review in ethics consultation. In: Finder SG, Bilton MJ (eds) Peer review, peer education, and modeling in the practice of clinical ethics consultation: the Zadeh project. Springer, Cham, pp 47–61
Hunter KM, Charon R, Coulehan JL (1995) The study of literature in medical education. Acad Med 70(9):787–794
Hurst SA, Chevrolet JC, Loew F (2006) Methods in clinical ethics: a time for eclectic pragmatism? Clin Ethics 1(3):159–164
Hynds J (2018) Ethics consultation, professional praxis, and what it means to be a "consultant". In: Finder SG, Bilton MJ (eds) Peer review, peer education, and modeling in the practice of clinical ethics consultation: the Zadeh project. Springer, Cham, pp 85–97
Jonsen AR (1991a) Casuistry as methodology in clinical ethics. Theor Med 12(4):295–307
Jonsen AR (1991b) Of balloons and bicycles – or – the relationship between ethical theory and practical judgment. Hastings Cent Rep 21(5):14–16
Jonsen AR (1995) Casuistry: an alternative or complement to principles? Kennedy Inst Ethics J 5(3):237–251
Jonsen AR, Siegler M, Winsdale WJ (2006) Clinical ethics: a practical approach to ethical decisions in clinical medicine, 6th edn. McGraw Hill, New York
Kopelman LM (1994) Case method and casuistry: the problem of bias. Theor Med 15(1):21–37
Kuczewski M (1998) Casuistry and Principlism: the convergence of method in biomedical ethics. Theor Med Bioeth 19(6):509–524
McCarthy J (2003) Principlism or narrative ethics: must we choose between them? Med Humanit 29(2):65–71
Miller FG, Fins JJ, Bacchetta MD (1996) Clinical pragmatism: John Dewey and Clinical ethics. J Contemp Health Law Policy 13(1):27–51
Rosell T, Johnson B (2018) This may, or may not, be an ethics consultation. In: Finder SG, Bilton MJ (eds) Peer review, peer education, and modeling in the practice of clinical ethics consultation: the Zadeh project. Springer, Cham, pp 99–107
Sugarman J, Sulmasy DP (2001) Methods in medical ethics, 1st edn. Georgetown University Press, Washington, DC
Tarzian AJ (2018) Ethics consultation for Mrs. Hamadani: a focus on process. In: Finder SG, Bilton MJ (eds) Peer review, peer education, and modeling in the practice of clinical ethics consultation: the Zadeh project. Springer, Cham, pp 75–84

(Meta-) Methodological Lessons for Ethics Consultation

Mark P. Aulisio

Introduction

At the outset of this chapter, I want to echo the praise offered by all of the contributors to this volume for Finder's outstanding, thoughtful and self-critical narrative of the case of 83 year old Mrs. Hamadani and her fiercely devoted children. The brocade account is carefully woven, like a fine Persian tapestry, to convey the rich complexity of an actual ethics consultation as it transpires not over hours, but rather over days, weeks, months and even, as in this case, years. Mrs. Hamadani's narrative so told is replete with questions worthy of critical reflection. What is an appropriate role for ethics consultation in healthcare? How can an autonomy-centric culture accommodate community-centric cultural difference? How can or should the voice of the patient be heard when she cannot speak for herself and the much louder and anguished voices of others demand to be heard? What are the bounds of acceptable medical treatment and how should care teams respond when patient or family demands threaten to push care givers to cross those bounds? What is an appropriate response for ethics consultants when they are asked to take over a case or prevent a colleague from interacting with an unwilling family? Do the motivations of patients, family, or members of the care team in calling ethics consultants necessarily shape the consultant's role? And so the list goes on, as the variety of commentaries which comprise the majority of this volume, as well as the multitude of discussions that you, the readers, will inevitably have with colleagues, students, and friends make abundantly clear.

Rather than attempting to answer any of these questions, my aim here will be suitably modest. That is, I hope to contribute to what will undoubtedly be an ongoing

M. P. Aulisio (✉)
Department of Bioethics, Case Western Reserve University School of Medicine, Cleveland, OH, USA
e-mail: mpa5@case.edu

S. G. Finder, M. J. Bliton (eds.), *Peer Review, Peer Education, and Modeling in the Practice of Clinical Ethics Consultation: The Zadeh Project*,
https://doi.org/10.1007/978-3-319-90955-4_9

conversation by offering a few reflections on the Hamadani case – reflections evoked by Finder's telling of Mrs. Hamadani's story – and their lessons for method in ethics consultation. These lessons might be better characterized as *meta*-methodological because they are at a level of generality that makes them, I think, compatible with and relevant for a wide variety of more specific models, approaches and methods for doing ethics consultation in healthcare settings. The reflections and their meta-methodological lessons concern underlying value conflict or uncertainty, decision-making authority, and focus of care.

Value Conflict or Uncertainty?

> "None of us thought she would live this long, and *Nadira and I have spent much of this time making sure that our mother is taken care of, that we do for her what she did for us, for all of us, even including our father, in the past.* Although I have lived here in the United States for almost 30 years, I still hold fast to some of the *values* that come from our homeland. And *respecting and caring for one's parents is high on the list. Unfortunately,"* and here she began to trail off, *"many here do not share this belief."* (Finder 2018: 32–3; emphasis added).

Thus Farzana Hamadani, the elder of the patient's two daughters, starkly articulates a difference in cultural *values* that, in her eyes, underlies so much of the struggle that she, her sister, Nadira, and brother, Samir Zadeh, have had in their nearly 4 year ordeal of caring for their mother, Mrs. Hamadani. Though she did not explicitly state it, it is clear from nature and number of conflicts with health professionals over these years that the struggle was often, in their eyes, made *more,* not less, difficult by the very people who were supposed to be *caring* for her mother. Indeed, we are told that upon Mrs. Hamadani's first admission to the hospital over 3 years earlier, a neurologist suggested hospice placement as a possibility for her only to be shouted out of the room, chased down the hall, and "fired" (Finder 2018: 22). At the time Mrs. Hamadani had newly diagnosed cancer, with metastases to her liver and brain, advanced Parkinson's, congestive heart failure, and renal insufficiency, making the hospice suggestion completely understandable. Despite this, the suggestion of hospice care was taken as disrespectful and uncaring, at worst, or callous, at best. Compounding the effrontery, the family believes that their mother has now had over 3 years with them and their father – years which surely she would not have had if they had not protected her from the uncaring neurologist.

At other points too, we are told, Mrs. Hamadani had need of the protection of her family *against* "care" providers; even on this admission. Samir in his impromptu first encounter with Finder relays,

> My mother, she is strong and after only a few days in the ICU she was well enough to go back to the floor. But the nurses there, they were not as attentive as the staff in the ICU, and my sister, Nadira, or our older sister, Farzana, or I would have to make sure they gave her medicines on time and that they fed her correctly. *Let me tell you Dr. Finder, we had to watch out or she would not get the care she needs to get stronger.* (Finder 2018: 24–5; emphasis added)

And

> *And then today, my mother was not doing so well, and it is, I believe, because they have not been giving her enough nutrition and so she is weak.* And she began to have difficulty breathing and she had to be emergently taken back to the ICU. (Finder 2018: 25; emphasis added)

As the family continues to protect Mrs. Hamadani from the care team, they become, true to Farzana's words, care-providers themselves. From feeding to removing the Bipap mask to carefully monitoring every health professional interaction with their mother, Samir, Farzana and Nadira continue to "respect and care" for her. The move from protector to active care-provider, even while Mrs. Hamadani is hospitalized, is a relatively short one. After all, if "many here" do not share the value of "respecting and caring for one's parents," how much less might they respect and care for another's parents?

Not surprisingly, the value difference underscored by Farzana in the passage quoted at the outset of this section is repeatedly echoed by Samir in his conversations with Finder and affirmed by Nadira and Farzana's behavior. From Samir's initial conversation about Finder's colleague, Dr. Moore, who was the first ethics consultant on the case, to his subsequent quasi-firing of Finder at the final family meeting there is tension about "respecting and caring for" one's parents:

> "But Dr. Finder," Mr. Zadeh continued, "your Dr. Moore, he has pestered us, always showing up when my mother has come into the hospital, asking us if we are ready to stop. *It's as if he doesn't know what it means to love your mother" … Mr. Zadeh's sister, Nadira, was gently wiping her eyes as Mr. Zadeh spoke.* (Finder 2018: 25; emphasis added)

> I do not want my mother to suffer, no one should ever want their mother to suffer. I do not need to hear 'we do not want your mother to suffer.' *What I want is for my mother to be taken care of, and when the time comes to make a decision, my sisters and I will decide, and we will do what is best for our mother … The doctors need to take care of my mother, the nurses need to do what they are supposed to do, and we, as the family, we will make the decisions that we need to make.* OK? (Finder 2018: 41; emphasis added)

Most of us would be quite taken aback, even offended, if we were told that "respecting and caring for one's parents" is not a value in our culture; more so if told it is not a value for us. Despite this, it is clear that this is precisely what Mrs. Hamadani's children believed both with respect to the broader cultural context and even more poignantly, that of healthcare. Given this belief, it is more than understandable that the Hamadani children would be compelled to stand watch, as sentinels, protecting her. A more plausible, and to most of us more palatable, explanation of the value laden cultural difference in the Hamadani case, however, is that the difference was less over the *value* of respecting and caring for one's parents and more over *what it means* to respect and care for ones parents, particularly in a healthcare context at a major medical center in the United States.

To unpack this a bit more, the two sides (a false binary but an easier way to speak of it) each interpreted differently what the values of "respecting and caring for" required in the case of Mrs. Hamadani. For members of the care team, respecting and caring for Mrs. Hamadani meant shifting the goals of care, sooner rather than later, to comfort; seeing to it that the dying process was shorter, rather than longer; and ensuring that Mrs. Hamadani was as free of pain and suffering as possible within the limits of acceptable medical practice. For the Hamadani family, respecting and caring for Mrs. Hamadani meant fighting disease as she was a "fighter" giving her as much "extra time" with them as she could have; directly providing care to her as they were able and as she had done for them for so many years; and keeping vigil until a decision was forced upon them.

If this analysis is correct, a deep value-laden difference about *what it meant to* "respect and care for" Mrs. Hamadani, and not about whether one *should* respect and care for her, was at the core of the Hamadani case. This difference was, to be sure, partly a function of culture, but I would suggest that it was also partly a function of the radically different role relationships of daughter or son, on the one hand, and healthcare professional, on the other. I suspect that this is one of the reasons this type of value conflict or uncertainty is sometimes present in cases in which there is no discernible cultural difference. Respecting and caring for one's *parent* and respecting and caring for one's *patient* need not, even stronger – *should not*, be the same. Mrs. Hamadani needed her devoted children caring for her as only children can, but she also needed devoted doctors, nurses, social workers, and care team members caring for her as their respective professional roles require. Early identification of differences in the meaning of "respecting and caring for" and analysis of its possible sources might have allowed those involved to better understand each other and move forward with less conflict. It might have also, over time, laid the groundwork for building a consensus among those involved to move forward in a way that may have made a difficult and burdensome case perhaps a little less so.

The first meta-methodological lesson from "The Zadeh Scenario," then, is that however one does ethics consultation, one of its core elements is to identify and analyze the nature of the values conflict or uncertainty that underlies the need for consultation.[1] Not explicitly doing this in the Hamadani case may be a methodological hazard of the heavily phenomenological approach so expertly employed by Finder (and presumably by Dr. Moore as well). While many of us no doubt fail to pay sufficient attention to the texture of the case as Finder does exceptionally well, it is also important to step back and abstract a bit from the concrete messiness and time pressures of the actual case to surface possible underlying issues, particularly those with important normative dimensions.

[1] Indeed, the first of two core features in ASBH's "ethics facilitation approach" is "to identify and analyze the nature of the value conflict or uncertainty underlying the consultation" (ASBH 1998, 2011; Aulisio et al. 2000). Elsewhere I have argued that ASBH's "Ethics Facilitation" approach is best understood as a more general normative characterization of ethics consultation that is informed by the context in which ethics consultation is done and is compatible with a wide variety of models and methodologies, among which is included phenomenological method as practiced by Dr. Finder and, presumably, Dr. Moore (Aulisio 2011). I should also add that not all cases that come to ethics consultation necessarily involve underlying value conflict or uncertainty, but helping to sort even this out is a valuable service.

Decision-Making Authority?

Above I suggested that a certain understanding of what it means to respect and care for one's parents along with familial and health professional role differences (at least partly) drove the Hamadani family to think that the value of respecting and caring for one's parents was somehow not shared by society in general or by members of the care team in particular. Such a belief makes very understandable their strong adoption of the protector and provider role on behalf of their mother. Just as protecting leads quickly and understandably to providing, "providing" leads quickly to "deciding." A recurring theme in "The Zadeh Scenario" as told by Finder is that there was an ongoing struggle, at least in the eyes of the Hamadani family, about decision-making. Interestingly, the struggle was not primarily about *who* would make decisions (except in one encounter), but rather about what decisions should be made and when they should be made.

Members of the care team, Drs. Moore and Finder, and the Hamadani family alike seem to be largely in agreement that the Hamadani children are the appropriate decision makers for Mrs. Hamadani. Disagreements emerge primarily over the content and timing of such decisions. For example, the first time decision-making is broached in the narrative, it is because members of the care team are concerned that Mrs. Hamadani's children are making "bad decisions" in their single minded determination to pursue aggressive, rather than comfort, care for Mrs. Hamadani (Finder 2018: 23). Similarly, when questions are raised about DNR status (an often contentious point between care team and family members) we are told time and again by members of the care team that the family is "not ready to make that kind of decision" (Finder 2018: 24; or the equivalent: 24, 26, 27, 28) or that they have put off a decision when approached by saying "now is not a good time" (multiple times; Finder 2018: 24, 28, 30, 31, 36, 40, 41).

To the extent that the Hamadani family had settled on anything, it appears that it was that they would pursue aggressive care as long as possible and make a decision about resuscitation (and all that it entails) only if their mother's heart stopped and such a decision was necessary. Dr. Broukhim's notes make this clear, as Finder writes:

> The notes for Mrs. Hamadani gave a very clear picture of all that had been going on, including his own assessment that Mrs. Hamadani was no longer a candidate for any kind of therapeutic interventions, that he had, since the beginning of this admission, been recommending a shift to a purely palliative focus, *that the family seemed to understand that their mother was likely near the end of her life, but that they also were, as of yet, unwilling to consent to anything less than full code and that they continued to ask about what other options might be considered.* (Finder 2018: 30; Broukhim note, emphasis added)

> With all of that in his note, what stood out next was that he then reported that "the family does not, at this time, wish to have me write a DNAR order, *that they prefer to wait until the decision to act must be made before giving permission not to proceed to intubation.*" (Finder 2018: 31; Broukhim note, emphasis added)

The repeated attempts to encourage the family to consider and decide on, first, comfort measures and, later, code status, are supported by Samir's comments to Finder as well. He describes Dr. Moore's "checking in" about decision-making as "pestering" and "always showing up when we come to the hospital asking us if we are ready to stop" (Finder 2018: 25). Samir is equally clear about *when* and *by whom* a decision to resuscitate will be made in his conversation with Dr. Finder, "And I told them that no decision like that needed to be made until her hearts stops; then we, my sisters and I, will decide what to do!" (Finder 2018: 25) and "we will decide whether to put her on machines" (Finder 2018: 26).

In my experience, the above internecine dynamic is far from rare. Family members feel badgered and pressured for "a decision" that is in line with the care team's recommendation, especially when comfort measures only or, at the very least, DNAR are being considered. They also often feel that they are not being heard and that members of the care team are approaching them the way Dr. Moore approached the family in Samir's eyes: "he simply came *to get us to say what he wanted to hear*" (Finder 2018: 26). Within this adversarial dynamic, that the family is the locus of decision-making or, more directly, that decision-making authority lies with the family is repeatedly affirmed and, ultimately, entrenched. Once entrenched, the struggle to "convince" the family commences. These struggles usually result in much collateral damage, not the least of which is the patient's voice cannot be heard above the din.

This internecine dynamic is set up by a mistake. The mistake is placing the locus of decision-making with the family. One of the fundamental normative features of our societal context, a context within which clinical ethics consultation is practiced, is that decision making authority for the once capacitated but now incapacitated patient rests squarely with the patient, i.e., the patient is the locus of decision-making. This is a function of a patient's right to live according to his or her own values, which values may have implications for medical decision-making (Aulisio 2003, 2014). Decision-making authority remains with Mrs. Hamadani, not with the care team or with the family. This is not to say that each of the latter do not have a role to play, far from it. The family's (surrogate's) role is to try to help make clear the values of the patient and what they might mean for decision-making.[2] The care team's role is, among other things, to articulate the range of medically acceptable options, as well as to be clear about their recommended option in the event that they have one.

The second meta-methodological lesson from "The Zadeh Scenario" is, then, that early on it is imperative that all concerned focus on the appropriate source for decision making authority and what that means for the role of family (surrogates) and care team in decision making. A good mechanism for ensuring such a focus is to hold a multidisciplinary team meeting followed by a family conference very early

[2]Elsewhere, I have argued that we should drop "decision-maker" when discussing the surrogate's role because it falsely connotes that surrogates are decision makers in a straightforward sense. This is, as I will discuss in the next section, confusing for health professionals and extremely burdensome for surrogates (Aulisio 2016).

in the patient's stay. This is not a panacea for difficult cases, as difficult cases will remain, well, difficult. Relative clarity about decision-making roles can, however, allow for more open lines of communication and, perhaps, serve as a prophylactic against the internecine dynamic characterized above.

Focus of Care?

My last reflection concerns a striking, albeit again all too common, feature of the Hamadani case. From Finder's narrative, it appears that as the case unfolded, the patient's family functionally became *the patient*, shifting not only the locus of decision-making but also the focus of care from Mrs. Hamadani to her devoted, but distressed and overburdened, children. This shift exacted a heavy toll from all concerned, most especially from the Hamadanis themselves.

Interestingly, there are no less than three points in the narrative when patient treatment decisions are made primarily *for the family's benefit* rather than the patient's. This constitutes what I would term the "family as patient" phenomenon. It first presents early in the narrative with Dr. Moore arranging for Broukhim to take over Mrs. Hamadani's care:

> *In an effort to help this family,* Steve was the one who had actually contacted Dr. Broukhim to see if he'd be willing to talk with Mr. Zadeh and his sisters; Broukhim had a reputation of being extremely aggressive—often too much so for some of the other physicians who frequently interacted with him—but he was beloved by his patients. (Finder 2018: 22–3)

The key here for our purposes is that Dr. Moore ("Steve") contacted Broukhim "in an effort to help this family" thinking that Broukhim would be very aggressive in accord with his reputation and consonant with the family's wishes.

A second instance of a patient care decision being made primarily for the benefit of the family occurs just over 3 years later. In Mrs. Hamadani's final stay, Steve reprises this role again by supporting the placement of an NG tube against Broukhim's advice, "In an effort to defuse this moment, Steve had offered that perhaps it would not be unreasonable to place the NG, since it offered little risk and only minimal discomfort given Mrs. Hamadani's state" (Finder 2018: 24). We are told that the "gamble… paid off in that Mr. Zadeh expressed appreciation to Steve for supporting *their* wishes for the NG" tube (Finder 2018: 24; emphasis added).

A third instance of treatment decisions being made primarily for the family's benefit occurs toward the end of the narrative and concerns the possibility of dialyzing Mrs. Hamadani. Despite the fact that the ICU attending (Dr. Smith), the consulting nephrologist (Dr. Nadouri) and Dr. Broukhim himself recommended against it, the family was insistent that dialysis be considered (Finder 2018: 31). In recounting Broukhim's note, Finder tells us

> Moreover, he reported a similar disposition regarding dialysis. And in the same breath (so to speak), he then wrote that he asked Dr. Nadouri to get a second renal consultant to take a look at Mrs. Hamadani in order to help determine if dialysis would be helpful. (Finder 2018: 31)

Thus, we are told that Dr. Broukhim agreed with the determination of the attending and the consulting nephrologist regarding the inappropriateness of dialysis but, nonetheless, requested that a second nephrologist be consulted solely, so far as we can tell, at the behest of the family. The day after reading Broukhim's detailed note on this matter, Finder met with him only to find out that the second nephrology consult (with Dr. Spector) yielded a very different result: Dr. Spector thought that a short trial of dialysis might be useful as it might address possible uremic encephalopathy (Finder 2018: 35) and thereby slightly improve mental status. To Finder's surprise, Broukhim accepted the assessment even though it was contrary to that of two other physicians and his own prior medical judgment. Furthermore, he queried Finder as to whether he thought a trial of dialysis would be reasonable. After some discussion, Broukhim offers the following conclusion,

> "I think with all that they've been through," Broukhim now said, "it's not unreasonable to see if we can wake her up *and give them a chance to have a little bit a final time together.* She's been a real fighter all along, and *they've been so involved in her care, I think I owe them this.*" (Finder 2018: 35; emphasis added)

The decision to dialyze Mrs. Hamadani had been made primarily, although not exclusively, for the benefit of her children.

These three examples of care decisions being made primarily for Mrs. Hamadani's children highlight what is, for me, a prominent theme in this powerful narrative.: somehow over the course of Mrs. Hamadani's 3-plus years after being diagnosed with metastatic cancer and her multiple admissions to the hospital, Mrs. Hamadani's children gradually became "the patient." Not only were they viewed as the source of decision making authority, they were also increasingly viewed as the proper subject of care, "the patient," in their own eyes and those of the care team. The narrative provides scores of examples of this. Indeed, at the conclusion of Finder's initial chance involvement with the family, Mr. Zadeh says to him,

> "You are a good listener, Dr. Finder, and I thank you. I believe you understand what it is like to face this sort of thing." And then he (Mr. Zadeh) said it: *"And so I beg of you, Doctor, please don't let Dr. Moore see my mother again. My sisters and I do not want him talking with us anymore."* (Finder 2018: 26; emphasis added)

And regarding this, Finder tells us,

> And for a second time since exiting the elevator and walking outside, I was taken aback somewhat. While there was a kind of forcefulness to Mr. Zadeh's request, as he spoke it, both he and his sister Nadira were both looking at me not with anger nor reproach, *but with eyes slightly wide and down-turned at the corners. I was struck by their sadness and apprehension, peppered with a bit of fear.* (Finder 2018: 26; emphasis added)

Mr. Zadeh's request to Dr. Finder that Dr. Moore no longer be involved in the case is fundamentally about the distress Moore's involvement is causing the family to experience. When Finder accedes to this request, he discovers upon visiting with Nadira and Farzana that the family is extremely appreciative of his having helped make "sure that Dr. Moore is no longer a bother" to them (Finder 2018: 32).

Interestingly, Dr. Broukhim in one of his notes makes clear that he personally asked Dr. Moore to stay involved in the case to, among other things, "provide as much support to the family" as he could (Finder 2018: 30). The family clearly did not feel supported by Dr. Moore as he, in the words of Mr. Zadeh, "did not *visit*, he simply came to get us to say what he wanted to hear" (Finder 2018: 26). Later, the family expresses appreciation to Dr. Finder for "visiting" with them (*contra* Moore) (Finder 2018: 34). In some ways Finder's role was really about being present to and "visiting" with those who are suffering – the patients – Mrs. Hamadani's children. Dr. Finder, like Dr. Moore before him, is ultimately, in a sense, fired from the case when his presence no longer eases the family's suffering and, perhaps, piques it when he shifts the focus again in his final comments to what is going to happen to Mrs. Hamadani and his concern that she not suffer:

> "You know, Dr. Finder," said Mr. Zadeh, "I think you are right. But the problem here is that everyone keeps telling me and my sisters all these bad things about what is going to happen to our mother as if we do not understand. But we do understand, we are not uneducated people. But is it too much to ask to please stop preaching about what is going to happen to our mother? We understand, we know, we get it!" His voice was now raised, and Farzana reached over as if to calm him, but he was in the grip of the moment, of release, perhaps. (Finder 2018: 41)

And later,

> He paused and then added, "Please Dr. Finder, I do not wish to cause problems, and I apologize for raising my voice. But I do not want to talk about this anymore and I do not want to talk with anyone else but Dr. Broukhim." (Finder 2018: 41)

Whether family, significant other, or friend, all those who deeply care about the patient are vulnerable, stressed, and burdened – they are suffering – and, as such, especially in a protracted case, they become *de facto* patients. They might be termed something like second order or secondary patients, because their suffering is largely a function of their concern for their loved one, the (first order or primary) patient. As family members et al. become *secondary* patients, *all involved run the risk of affording them the status of (primary) patients with potentially devastating consequences.* That status includes many of the features of the Hamadani case as discussed above, not the least of which is that family members become *the* decision makers (as if they were the patient) and treatment decisions start to be made primarily out of concern for the impact on the family and in accord with the family's concerns rather than patient values.

The empirical literature is now filled with examples of the heavy burdens shouldered by surrogate decision-makers (see, for example, Wendler and Rid 2011). The growing literature on surrogate decision making underscores the severe nature of this burden. In a study of family members of 294 ICU patients, for example, 33.1% of all family members exhibited symptoms consistent with moderate to major risk of developing Post-Traumatic Stress Disorder (Azoulay et al. 2005). The percentage jumped to 47.8% for family members who "shared in decision making" and a stunning 81.8% for family members who "shared in end of life decisions." Another study of 30 surrogates in five ICUs found that surrogates experience "significant emotional conflict between the desire to act in accordance with their loved one's values and 1) not wanting to feel responsible for a loved one's death, 2) a desire to pursue any chance of recovery, and 3) the need to preserve family well-being" (Schenker et al. 2012). From the narrative, there can be little doubt that Samir, Nadira, and Farzana experienced significant emotional conflict about competing concerns and likely exhibited symptoms of Post-Traumatic Stress Disorder as well.

The third and final meta-methodological point is that many of the cases brought to ethics consultation will inevitably involve families or loved ones who are secondary patients. All of us who perform clinical ethics consultation need to be careful that the patient's family or loved one's do not functionally become *the (primary) patient*, shifting not only the locus of decision-making but also the focus of care as appeared to happen in the Hamadani case. In order to avoid this, we have to acknowledge the emotional needs of family members and loved ones, marshaling all support resources at our disposal (pastoral care ministry, social work, bereavement groups, counseling services, etc.) to attend to those needs. In addition, as I have argued above and elsewhere, we need to work to make clear early on that patients, not family members, other surrogates or even health professionals, are the locus of decision-making authority in our societal context due to the rights of individuals to live by their own values. In a real sense, once capacitated but now incapacitated patients remain the decision makers with the rest of us playing a support role in seeing to it that any decisions made reflect those values within the bounds of medically appropriate care. Taking this normative feature of our societal context seriously means we should not approach family members or loved ones for a "decision" or "consent" or ask "what do you want us to do?" We should, rather, frame issues over and against clearly articulated surrogate, team member and patient roles in which, whatever else is entailed, the patient is accepted as the clear source of decision making authority and focus of care.

References

American Society for Bioethics and Humanities (1998) Core competencies for health care ethics consultation: the report of the American Society for Bioethics and Humanities, 1st edn. ASBH, American Society for Bioethics and Humanities, Glenview, pp 3–10

American Society for Bioethics and Humanities (2011) Core competencies for health care ethics consultation: the report of the American Society for Bioethics and Humanities, 2nd edn. ASBH, American Society for Bioethics and Humanities, Glenview, pp 2–10

Aulisio MP (2003) Meeting the need: ethics consultation in health care today. In: Aulisio MP, Arnold RM, Youngner SJ (eds) Ethics consultation: from theory to practice. Johns Hopkins University Press, Baltimore, pp 1–22

Aulisio MP (2011) "Facilitated consensus," "ethics facilitation," and unsettled cases. J Clin Ethics 22(4):345–353 author reply 358-362

Aulisio MP (2014) Advance directives and the physician-patient relationship: a surprising metamorphosis. In: Lack P, Biller-Adorno N, Brauer S (eds) Advance directive. Springer, Dordrecht, pp 127–152

Aulisio M (2016) "So what do you want us to do?" Patients' rights, unintended consequences, and the Surrogate's role. Oxford Handbooks Online. Retrieved 23 Jan. 2016, from http://www.oxfordhandbooks.com/view/10.1093/oxfordhb/9780199974412.001.0001/oxfordhb-9780199974412-e-13

Aulisio MP, Arnold RM, Youngner SJ (2000) Health care ethics consultation: nature, goals, and competencies. A position paper from the Society for Health and Human Values-Society for Bioethics Consultation Task Force on Standards for Bioethics Consultation. Ann Intern Med 133(1):59–69

Azoulay E, Pochard F, Kentish-Barnes N et al (2005) Risk of post traumatic stress symptoms in family members of intensive care unit patients. Am J Respir Crit Care Med 171(9):987–994

Finder SG (2018) The Zadeh scenario. In: Finder SG, Bliton MJ (eds) Peer review, peer education, and modeling in the practice of clinical ethics consultation: the Zadeh project. Springer, Cham, pp 21–42

Schenker Y, Crowley-Matoka M, Dohan D, Tiver GA, Arnold RM, White DB (2012) I don't want to be the one saying 'we should just let him die': intrapersonal tensions experienced by surrogate decision makers in the ICU. JGIM 27(12):1657–1665

Wendler D, Rid A (2011) Systematic review: the effect on surrogates of making treatment decisions for others. Ann Intern Med 154(5):336–346

Narrative and Method in Ethics Consultation

George J. Agich

Introduction

Method in ethics consultation has at least three distinguishable components: a canon, a discipline, and a history (Agich 2001). The term *canon* refers to the set of rules that guides the actions, cognitions, judgments, and perceptions involved in performing an ethics consultation. Because ethics consultation is a practice and not just a body of knowledge, the *rules* in ethics consultation are best thought of as the internal normative aspects of the actions that make up an ethics consultation. In a practice, the term *rule has* a special meaning. In a practice, rules are *enacted. Practice* is a technical term that was introduced into bioethics by Alasdair MacIntyre in his well-known book, *After Virtue*:

> A practice may be identified as a set of considerations, manners, uses, observances, customs, standards, canons, maxims, principles, rules and offices specifying useful procedures or denoting obligations or duties which relate to human actions and utterances. It is … an adverbial qualification of choices and performances, more or less complicated in which conduct is understood in terms of a procedure. Words such as punctually, considerately, civilly, scientifically, legally, candidly, judicially, poetically, morally, etc., do not specify performances; they postulate performances and specify *procedural conditions* to be taken into account when choosing and acting. (MacIntyre 1981: 55–6, emphasis added)

In the practice of doing ethics consultation, the rules are embedded in the practical actions and intentions of those performing ethics consultations. Some rules, of course, are articulated and even expressed formulaically. Slowther et al. report in a national study of clinical ethics services in the UK that

> When asked about the use of decision-making frameworks, over half of the responders to this question (28/50, 56%) reported using the 'four principles' approach in the previous

G. J. Agich (✉)
Bowling Green State University, Bowling Green, OH, USA
e-mail: agichg@bgsu.edu

S. G. Finder, M. J. Bliton (eds.), *Peer Review, Peer Education, and Modeling in the Practice of Clinical Ethics Consultation: The Zadeh Project*,
https://doi.org/10.1007/978-3-319-90955-4_10

> 12 months. Other less commonly used frameworks were the Ethox approach (18/50, 36%), the Four Quadrant approach (5/50, 10%) and the Dilemma method (3/50, 6%). Some used more than one framework and 15/50 (30%) said that they did not use any. (Slowther et al. 2012: 212)

These findings, however, do not tell us how these frameworks function as rules that actually guide ethics consultants as they engage in the doing of doing ethics consultation. In fact, this finding only focuses on decision-making frameworks and gives no insight into the myriad of other rules embedded in what consultants actually engaged in as they perform ethics consultations. Nonetheless, this is a good example of the plethora of articulated rules for ethics consultation. Similarly, the rules and procedures in conflict resolution or arbitration approaches can be articulated, but they must be acquired and put into practice. That is why experience is essential for competent ethics consultation since rules can be enacted only through practice.

The term *discipline* of ethics consultation refers to the mastery, or at least possession, of the specific types of actions and intentions of ethics consultants which are guided by the rules that are embodied in the actions of competent ethics consultants. The discipline of ethics consultation importantly includes specific training/experience through which the consultant develops the requisite capacities for performing ethics consultation in a competent fashion. In this sense, ethics consultation as a discipline is constituted in practice and can be thought of as having a particular set of meanings that makes it a distinctive way of engaging in patient care. Although sharing family resemblances with other clinical consultations that occur in the course of patient care, ethics consultation has and is a unique discipline. Its purposes, actions, and range of outcomes are distinct and unique to ethics consultation as opposed to other clinical consultations.

The term *history* refers to the narrative of the actions, including the analyses, assessments, and communications undertaken in the course of the consultation; it also importantly includes reasoning about the practical issues and the steps toward resolving the ethical question or issues that arose. The various key actions, perceptions, and judgments of the consultant and others involved in the case are told or recorded. In the fullest sense, this would include any medical record notes made by the ethics consultant(s), the ethics consultation service case records of the case, and any personal narrative(s) of the case by the involved consultants. History, as an aspect of method, also includes the development of both the competence of individual ethics consultants or consultation services and the field as a whole (McCullough 2001). Any defensible history of ethics consultation should include the actual reasoning employed or reflection about not only the actions or processes followed by the consultants, but the values and norms which motivated the ethics consultant in undertaking the actions performed. Explanation of and the justification for the actions and recommendations of the ethics consultant may not always be communicated fully in the medical record notes, but should be at least documented in summary fashion within internal ethics consultation service records and should be discussed in consultation case reviews. In this sense, the *history* of ethics consultation is not simply a set of narratives or stories about cases, but rather is, ideally, a set of critical reflections on both the actions and communications of ethics consultants in the course of doing the consultation and the decisions made or recommendations offered. The latter are often the primary focus of the discussion and review of ethics consultation reports or narratives clinical ethics cases, for example, in the course of ethics committee reviews as well as in the literature on clinical ethics cases. This focus on decision-making or recommendations, however, is unfortunate insofar as it tends to minimize the importance of the constituent actions and intentions that make up the process of doing clinical ethics consultations. The processes followed shape the case as it proceeds, and a good history captures this.

Critical reflection on the actions and communications involved in doing ethics consultation is essential not only in retrospective review of cases, but also in the process of actually performing an ethics consultation. I have argued that ethics consultation is best understood as a reflective practice and that the ethics consultant should be a reflective practitioner who is intentionally aware of and responsible for the actions and communications routinely undertaken in the course of an ethics consultation (Agich 2015; Schön 1983). These actions and communications include the phases of gathering information, assessment, interpretation, deciding which clinicians should be interviewed, when and how interviews and/or meetings should be conducted, as well as which individuals should be involved in the meetings. These actions, of course, are not undertaken in a linear fashion, but are adjusted to the particular circumstances of the case and are recursive, in the sense that they are often repeated. Thus, the phases of ethics consultation should not be conceived as a standardized or formal structure, but they are rather distinguishable aspects of what ethics consultants actually do in the course of their work. The ideal of ethics consultant as a reflective practitioner implies that competent ethics consultants will consciously and reflectively as well as responsibly engage in the component actions and engagements that compose an ethics consultation (Agich 2005: 14).

These points are not so much points in a *theory* of method in ethics consultation as a *description* of the key elements of what method *is* in the "doings" of ethics consultation. These points constitute a description of how ethics consultation is phenomenologically displayed if one makes a concerted effort to neutrally describe its essential features along a wide range of cases. As a doing, ethics consultation consists in actions and intentions that constitute a distinctive set of meanings in the clinical space of patient care (Agich 2005, 2009a). The meanings brought to patient care through the actions and communications of the ethics consultant shape to some extent the way that the case develops, though this can vary significantly depending on the actual circumstances of the case and the issues at hand. Hopefully, these meanings and interpretations as well as reflections are communicated in narratives about the case.

Method as the Lens to View the Field of Clinical Ethics

How does this characterization of method in ethics consultation as a practice help us to understanding the field? First, the underlying concept of a practice requires us to focus on the actual "doings," e.g., the actions, cognitions and perceptions of ethics consultants actually engaging in consultation. Second, viewing ethics consultation as a practice has the important implication that the question of method has to be regarded as a practical, and not a theoretical, matter. The rules involved in ethics consultation are first and foremost enacted and are phenomenologically manifested in and through the actions, cognitions, and perceptions of consultants. The rules are not and cannot be reduced to a formal code or set of guidelines or procedures that might be followed like a recipe. Instead, the rules, even when articulated linguistically, as they certainly must be for various legitimate purposes, are just abstractions from the lived experience of the practice and, importantly, they are dependent upon that practice for their ultimate meaning and justification. In this sense, statements about ethics consultation methodology, and theories of ethics consultation, are *secondary* to the actual practice itself.

Formal statements of rules of practice, of course, have a purpose. They permit individuals without directly relevant experience in doing the actual consultation to have meaningful discussions about it and they can have proactive effect in shaping the actual doings of ethics consultants. So, for example, understanding patient autonomy and patient rights, the right to information and to personal medical decision-making, provide a normative, conceptual framework for undertaking actions such as directly communicating with patients or their surrogates rather than relying upon the statements or reports of health professionals. But simply *knowing* or *understanding* the concepts of autonomy and medical decision-making does nothing to provide the communicative, interpretive, and decisional skills that are exercised by consultants actually engaged in ethics consultations as they go about respecting patient autonomy. These skills, the putting into action, as it were, of the ethical and legal concepts of patient rights are acquired and developed through the experience of actually performing ethics consultations – and not through knowledge as such. In other words, the knowledge of any doing or practice is properly and primarily expressed in the doings themselves, the actions that make up the practice. Like all practical activities, competence in ethics consultation is fundamentally acquired through experience, through learning and repetition, and not primarily through cognitive or intellectual learning. For novices in ethics consultation, the articulated rules or guidelines can help, but experienced ethics consultants, like experienced practitioners in any field, operate with rules in the background as it were. The rules come to be embodied and habituated in the actions of competent ethics consultants as they do in competent practitioners in any field.

In this sense, the rules of ethics consultation can be thought of as performative. In the philosophy of language, J. L. Austin introduced the concept of a *performative* as a distinctive type of speech act (Austin 1962). The uttering of a performative is, or is part of, the doing of a certain kind of action, the performance of which is not just a "saying" or "describing" something, but essentially a doing (Austin 1962: 5). Whereas Austin was primarily concerned with speech acts as a mainly linguistic phenomenon, ethics consultation involves not just pronouncements as such might be articulated in a recommendation at the end of an ethics consultation, but in various other communications and actions. Since ethics consultation involves complex analysis, interpretation, communication, as well as reflection on the information associated with the clinical case, performative speech acts in Austin's sense is only one component. Even with respect to speech acts alone, I tend to agree with Bach and Harnish (1979), who claimed that performatives are successful only if recipients infer the intention behind the literal meaning. So, when regarded solely as speech acts, performatives are acts of the social phenomenon and process of communication and involve the social construction of meaning. Even performative speech acts such as "I pronounce you man and wife" succeed not by conformity to convention as Austin seems to have it, but by the recognition by and acceptance by others of the intention of the person who does the communicating. The occasion of the marriage ceremony in which the pronouncement is articulated by a duly constituted official is itself a social construction with a frame of meanings. These meanings are enmeshed in these social frameworks. The success of performative speech acts as communication thus depends not only on an audience to identify the speaker's intention and, in an important sense, to accept it, but also to understand and accept the background normative framework for the recommendations.

Despite the limitations mentioned, the linguistic concept of performative utterances is helpful to make an important point about ethics consultation, namely that as a practice ethics consultation essentially *is* nothing more than the various actions that constitute the meanings of the individuals involved in performing the ethics consultation. As ethics consultation services have become accepted in healthcare institutions, the consultations in many places take on a ceremonial aspect. In some, there is the ceremony of the family meeting or the healthcare team meeting in which crucial discussions occur and decisions are made. In other settings, ethics consultations are performed along the lines of clinical consultations by individual consultants or teams to function independently in the consultative capacity and independently make judgments about whether team meetings or family meetings are appropriate. In either approach, the meaningfulness of statements made in the course of ethics consultation are therefore fundamentally dependent upon the wider set of social meanings that provide a framework of acceptance of the particular doings of ethics consultants by patients, families, and health professionals (Agich 1995, 2000). This dependence can, however, become an uncritical habit or tradition that can function and be invoked unreflectively to justify recommendations or decisions. Such a routinization of actions—and justifications in ethics consultation—and their acceptance by the "audience" of patients/families and health professionals, thus poses the danger that ethics consultation will itself become routine and occur without significant critical reflection. I will return to this point when I discuss the Zadeh Scenario in a moment.

To summarize, the question of method of ethics consultation is fundamentally tied to the complex construction or constitution of the social reality of ethics consultation in the clinical care of patients. Unlike performative utterances, which are mere speech acts, ethics consultation is much more complex in that it involves a performance that includes not just distinctive performative communications (as in the decision-making or the making of recommendations by ethics consultants, which are so often the focus of much discussion of clinical ethics cases) but also the constitution of meanings which comprises the interpretation and analysis of the clinical ethical circumstances of the case by the ethics consultant. The analysis and interpretation of actions and communications of those involved in the clinical care of the patient is thus a complex process that melds the meaning of ethical concepts, principles, and theories with the constructed and uncovered clinical and value meanings of the case.

Method as a Lens to View Cases: The Zadeh Example

That said, how a case is understood and represented does disclose a great deal about the adequacy of the processes, namely the actions and communications, that make up an ethics consultation. Assessment and analysis of the way a case or clinical problem is presented is one foremost responsibility of ethics consultants and consultation services. Unless they fully accept this responsibility and act accordingly, their role will lack that structure and purpose that is central to the method of ethics consultation (Agich 2009b). The rules of the practice of ethics consultation are normatively framed in terms of helping to achieve an ethically justified outcome in a case. This is accomplished by providing advice on the ethical problems, confusions, conflicts, and questions that arise in the course of patient care. Defining what are the appropriate and defensible *ethical* concerns and distinguishing them from other concerns involved in patient care is rightly recognized as a central competence of ethics consultants (ASBH 2011: 12). Otherwise, consultants will function less as independent professionals and independent moral agents than as functionaries for others: health professionals or family members. If this happens, their role will shift from performing an *ethics* consultation to providing some other service such as emotional support. Providing emotional support, of course, is not unimportant in ethics consultation, but it is not the primary function of a competent ethics consultant. In ethics consultation, the primary function is to provide analysis and advice of the ethical and value concerns raised in the case. The primary focus should be the concerns relating directly to the ethically best course of care for the particular patient, but other important concerns such as supporting the family or health care providers as they deal with the stresses involved in the case should be ancillary. In cases where the decision-making legitimately falls to surrogates, because the patient lacks decisional capacity which has been appropriately assessed, then providing emotional support for the surrogates becomes more important, but it is still secondary to addressing the ethical concerns and questions arising in the case.

How do these points on method help us to understand "The Zadeh Scenario"? Although I concur with the observations and criticisms so well-articulated by Frolic and Rubin (2018), Armstrong (2018), Tarzian (2018), Hynds (2018), and Rosell and Johnson (2018) that "The Zadeh Scenario" raises deep questions about the role, including the specific actions, of the consultants involved, as well as normative questions, I will not pursue them deeply. Suffice it to say that it is troubling that the narrative omits mention, much less critical discussion, of the patient's wishes and values or reference to the ethical, legal, healthcare institutional policy, or professional guidelines which emphasize *patient* rights and should provide guidance about the responsibilities and limitations of the role of surrogates, family or otherwise. Also, no mention is made of the existence of an advance directive or discussions with the patient when she was functional about her preferences and values. Instead, the focus throughout is on decisions about specific medical interventions that are simply *presumed* to be within the legitimate and, indeed, the sole purview of the patient's family rather than the patient herself or even, it seems at points, of the physicians. These omissions are troubling. Since the form of this narrative is not a formal ethics consultation report, it is hard to judge whether these concerns were ever addressed in the course of the actual consultation or were simply omitted from the narrative, so I will leave them aside. Pointing out these concerns, however, raises a question about the purpose and nature of "The Zadeh Scenario," which affects how to approach it. Is it a narrative of an ethics consultation *as an ethics consultation* or rather a narrative of events and recollections about a long-running set of involvements with a particular set of family members, and health professional to a lesser extent, that occurred for a particular ethics consultant? There may be other alternatives, of course.

Given my focus on method, I will discuss some of the elements of the narrative that reveal the method used or as it is reported in the consultation, rather than dwell further on the more substantive matters. My focus is thus primarily on process aspects, such as communication among the consultants and the use of ethics consultation records, since these are the most prominent in the narrative. In the case of the narrator, Finder, we have his direct statements about some of his thoughts and actions, which we accept at face value, but in the case of his colleague, Steve Moore, we only have Finder's report and no direct report by Moore of his actions and intentions. With these limitations in mind, we can nonetheless ask what methodological features stand out.

There are four that I will discuss: first, timely and direct communication among members of the ethics consultation service regarding on going cases, i.e., in this case Drs. Moore and Finder, who are the only ones identified; second, written ethics consultation notes and records; third, the role projected by the ethics consultants through their actions and communications in the case; and fourth, the dynamic character of ethics consultations, which is most evident in complex and protracted consultations.

First, Finder's narrative provides a wonderful example of effective timely and direct communication among members of an ethics consultation service regarding on going cases. Although the consultation model demonstrated in this narrative is the individual consultant, effective and timely communication among members of ethics consultation teams or even committees in concurrent consultation is equally important. In this narrative, communication is reported to have occurred through the use of records of various sorts, including the electronic medical record and, presumably, of ethics consultation service records that it appears Finder reviewed at points and added to. The communication among the ethics consultants in this narrative is especially effective, because although Moore was directly involved over a long period of time, Finder was remarkably aware of many of the salient features of this involvement and details of the case. This included not only the content, but the tone and style of communications that Moore had with family members and other health professionals. Communication among ethics consultation service members is essential. Face-to-face oral communication and discussion about on-going cases is ideal, though not likely to occur regularly, such as in a team consultation settings in which members rotate. For this reason and because memory is not always reliable, as Finder noted at one point where he states that he wanted to write down his thoughts while they were fresh, good consultation service records are important. They can take many forms and a discussion of these forms is beyond the scope here.

However, consultation service records should include relevant factual data such as names and other identifying information of individuals involved, dates of service and a summary of the interactions with individuals, a summary of discussions, and impressions and interpretations that guide the consultant. Ideally, ethics consultation service records should include also some reflection on the normative guidelines relied upon and ethical analysis as it occurs in the case of the information encountered and the ethical justification or explanation of the actions, including recommendations made by the consultant. Such an ideal ethics consultation record would provide not only a summary set of statements of the encounters and actions that make up any ethics consultation, though each might be disconnected of course by the temporally discrete character of a case as it develops, but it should also include reflection on the individual instances of analytical, interpretive, reflective, and communicative actions that constitute the process of doing ethics consultation. Ethics consultation service records that primarily focus on recommendations made and the clinical circumstances or facts underlying those recommendations are, quite frankly, less useful and less likely to contribute to the development of a reflective practice, which I have argued should be the ideal for ethics consultation (Agich 2015).

Second, as already noted above, the narrative makes clear the importance of having and using written ethics consultations notes and records for ongoing ethics consultations. Such records are essential for quality improvement. They can provide a basis for peer review of the actual processes that make up complex ethics consultations and provide opportunities for reflections on how to improve existing practices. Having a record of the specific ways that individual ethics consultants attend to the questions or issues can point to differences in approach, which can be useful guides for ways to improve the overall practice of the consultation service. If the consultation service records only (or primarily) include documentation of case-related decisions, recommendations, or their explanations and justifications, it will be easier to miss those component actions that constitute and frame these outcomes. The importance of this point is easiest to see if one considers how one gains confidence and experience in any practical endeavor. Focusing on the outcome, the product produced, for example, by a craftsman cannot show the actual methods, the processes and procedures, and the underlying capacities and skills used to generate the result in question. To be able to effectively implement quality improvement in ethics consultation services' purposes, the review of cases must include critical discussion, reflection, and analysis of the processes and procedures undertaken by consultants as they do their work.

Third, the role that ethics consultants projects through their actions and communications is aptly illustrated in this narrative. Whether "The Zadeh Scenario" is an accurate or, rather, a full portrayal of the actions and communications we do not know, but taken at face value it is clear that several important normative ethical considerations are strikingly absent from this narrative. Instead, we have a picture of ethics consultants who seem to understand and so enact their primary role as that of providing "support," though it is never made clear how "support" is understood. What is provided is not just supportive listening to family members or emotional counseling, but making and reinforcing decisions about medical care that solidify the prerogatives of family members to make decisions. Since there is no discussion of patient wishes or of any deep exploration of patient values except as marginally provided by family members, the role that is projected in this narration is that of a sensitive communicator and counselor for family and, to some extent, health professionals, but not of individuals who are engaged in what might typically be called an *ethics* consultation. I say "to some extent," because the salient issue of moral distress of health professionals involved in this case over time is sidestepped in this narrative. This raises important issues about the usefulness of "The Zadeh Scenario" as a model for revealing how normative ethical considerations guide methodological choices made in doing ethics consultation, but, again, discussing that more fully is a concern beyond the scope of the present chapter.

Fourth, this narrative admirably demonstrates the dynamic character of ethics consultation. Not all ethics cases develop over long periods of time, but even within rather straightforward consultations there are episodes, such a receiving the request, validating or interpreting the issues or questions raised in the request, etc., that have specific structures and within which various actions and intentions of the consultants are displayed. The purpose of good or comprehensive ethics consultation records, whatever their form, is that the processes followed by the consultants in the case as it develops over time are recorded and able to be analyzed. Since ethics consultants perform multiple kinds of actions, good records capture and express these actions and interpretations within the broad set of social interactions of multiple individuals involved in the case as they evolve over time. The dynamic character of ethics consultations is, of course, most evident in complex and protracted consultations that bring ethics consultants together with patients, family members, and health professionals over longer periods of time. But, even in straightforward ethics consultations involving, for example, providing a reminder or information about the applicability of a hospital policy to a case, the question or issue that is raised occurs at a particular time in the course of the care of a particular patient and the question or issue is raised by a particular individual involved in the case. Even in dealing with straightforward ethical questions or issues, ethics consultants thus step into and act as agents in patient care at particular point in the case's development. The point of entry, though not much discussed, can affect how the consultant functions and whether the consultant is able to function effectively as an *ethics* consultant.

Conclusion

The dynamic character of clinical ethics cases is not surprising given the highly dynamic character of patient care, especially the care of patients who are seriously ill. This means that a substantial amount of information relevant to the ethical analysis of the case such as clinical data, no matter how seemingly straightforward, always have a timestamp and can expire quite quickly as circumstances change. Interpretations of data and clinical findings not only evolve over time, but are often diverse. Attending physicians, consultants, and other involved health professionals, not to mention multiple family members, can have different and even divergent understandings of the same "facts." This complicates the communicative process inordinately and can be one of the subtle points of divergence of opinion that is a source of conflict. Because ethics consultation typically occurs in the course of patient care in healthcare institutions which are also inherently complex, involving multiple healthcare professionals interacting over time and across shifts, ethical assessment must be recursive.

Moreover, good communication and reflection on that communication is a fundamental prerequisite for ethics consultants involved in a case. This means that as the patient's medical condition develops over time and as changes occur in healthcare personnel caring for patient and in the involvement of various members of the patient's family, the consultant must constantly reappraise and redefine the ethical problems and challenges. In the latter case, the family of a patient present at the bedside may cycle through multiple individuals, which complicates communication and decision-making for all involved. This fluid character of patient care underscores the importance of critical reflection by ethics practitioners on an ethics consultation service in ongoing cases. When this reflection is weak or omitted, the involvement of the consultant loses focus on the primary ethical responsibilities associated with ethics consultation.

In this commentary, I have focused on the question of method in ethics consultation and outlined its salient features stressing the point throughout that ethics consultation should be a reflective practice. It is important to note that "The Zadeh Scenario" provides detailed description of the actions, communications, and reflections by Finder on his involvement in the case; it also includes statements about the actions and involvements of Moore. However, this narrative seriously omits critical reflection on normative aspects of the case or the purpose of the consultation as an ethics consultation. This appears to be at the bottom of what bothers each of the peer reviewers. Although "The Zadeh Scenario" does not provide a strong exemplar of critical reflection on ethics consultation, we cannot conclude that it did not occur. Its absence in the narrative, however, raises significant questions about the adequacy of this form of narrative as a narrative *of an ethics consultation* from which we can gain understanding and gain greater insight into how to improve our practices. That being said, the narrative does serve as a very useful occasion to reflect on the nature of method in ethics consultation.

References

Agich GJ (1995) Authority in ethics consultation. J Law Med Ethics 23:273–283

Agich GJ (2000) Why should anyone listen to ethics consultants? In: Engelhardt HT (ed) The philosophy of medicine. Kluwer Academic Publishers, Dordrecht/Boston, pp 117–137

Agich GJ (2001) The question of method in ethics consultation. AJOB 1(4):31–41

Agich GJ (2005) What kind of doing is ethics consultation? Theor Med Bioeth 26(1):7–24

Agich GJ (2009a) Clinical ethics as practice. J Int Bioethique 20(4):15–24

Agich GJ (2009b) Why quality is addressed so rarely in clinical ethics consultation. Camb Q Healthc Ethics 18(4):333–337

Agich GJ (2015) Diversity in clinical ethics. In: Rassmussen LM, Iltis AS, Cherry MJ (eds) At the foundations of bioethics and biopolitics: critical essays on the thought of H Tristram Engelhardt, Jr. Springer, Cham, pp 13–33

American Society for Bioethics and Humanities (2011) Core competencies for healthcare ethics consultation, 2nd edn. American Society for Bioethics and Humanities, Glenview

Armstrong K (2018) Telling about engagement is not enough: seeking the "ethics" of Ethics Consultation in Clinical Ethics Case Reports. In: Finder SG, Bliton MJ (eds) Peer review, peer education, and modeling in the practice of clinical ethics consultation: the Zadeh project. Springer, Cham, pp 63–73

Austin JL (1962) How to do things with words. Clarendon Press, Oxford

Bach K, Harnish RM (1979) Linguistic communication and speech acts. MIT Press, Cambridge, MA

Finder SG (2018) The Zadeh scenario. In: Finder SG, Bliton MJ (eds) Peer review, peer education, and modeling in the practice of clinical ethics consultation: the Zadeh project. Springer, Cham, pp 21–42

Frolic A, Rubin SB (2018) Critical self-reflection as moral practice: a collaborative meditation on peer review in ethics consultation. In: Finder SG, Bliton MJ (eds) Peer review, peer education, and modeling in the practice of clinical ethics consultation: the Zadeh project. Springer, Cham, pp 47–61

Hynds J (2018) Ethics consultation, professional praxis, and what it means to be a "consultant". In: Finder SG, Bliton MJ (eds) Peer review, peer education, and modeling in the practice of clinical ethics consultation: the Zadeh project. Springer, Cham, pp 85–97

Macintyre A (1981) After virtue. University of Notre Dame Press, South Bend

McCullough LB (2001) The history of medical ethics is crucial for a critical perspective in the continuing development of ethics consultation. AJOB 1(4):55–57

Rosell T, Johnson B (2018) This may, or may not, be an ethics consultation. In: Finder SG, Bliton MJ (eds) Peer review, peer education, and modeling in the practice of clinical ethics consultation: the Zadeh project. Springer, Cham, pp 99–107

Schön D (1983) The reflective practitioner: how professionals think in action. Basic Books, New York

Slowther AM, McClimans L, Price C (2012) Development of clinical ethics services in the UK: a national survey. J Med Ethics 38(4):210–214

Tarzia AJ (2018) Ethics consultation for Mrs. Hamadani: a focus on process. In: Finder SG, Bliton MJ (eds) Peer review, peer education, and modeling in the practice of clinical ethics consultation: the Zadeh project. Springer, Cham, pp 75–84

Standardizing the Case Narrative

Lisa Rasmussen

Introduction

This chapter is a meta-commentary on case commentaries, in which theoretical questions about method in clinical ethics consultation meet the concrete exigencies of the practice. The difficulty in this task is looking through the lens of a case narrative that is necessarily limited (because it is a distillation of an experience lived through days and weeks of interaction with many people), and a set of commentaries that are themselves limited. The view this perspective may give of a consultation is not the same as the view that might result from an observer accompanying a consultant throughout the case. For example, commenters in this volume uniformly note additional information that was not provided in an already long case narrative. We have no evidence about whether these issues were broached in the case consultation itself; what we *do* know is that these issues did not appear in the narrative. As a result, this is a book about narrative composition as much as it is about methods in clinical ethics consultation.

But questioning narrative composition of consultation summaries does generate profitable discussion about the field of clinical ethics consultation itself. As we move towards standardization and quality improvement in clinical ethics consultation, peer review is a vital component for evaluating consultants and consultations. In this, we are hampered by the fact that there is no sustainable mechanism for allowing peer review of full consultations, and even less chance of observing a single consultant's practice over many cases. Instead, we have the proxy (as currently utilized in the Attestation model [Kodish et al. 2013]) of the consultant's case study. A flaw in this model is the possibility that excellent consultants can be poor writers, and that gifted writers may be poor consultants (where by "gifted" and "poor"

L. Rasmussen (✉)
University of North Carolina – Charlotte, Charlotte, NC, USA
e-mail: lrasmuss@uncc.edu

S. G. Finder, M. J. Bliton (eds.), *Peer Review, Peer Education, and Modeling in the Practice of Clinical Ethics Consultation: The Zadeh Project*,
https://doi.org/10.1007/978-3-319-90955-4_11

writing I am referring to narrative compositional choices in addition to word or style choices). If we are to be evaluated by our case narratives, we must try to control for features irrelevant to quality evaluation, such as narrative ability, rhetorical skill and seductive rococo vocabulary.[1]

We may also want to control for the consultant's perspective: What we choose to accent in a narrative is what is important or noteworthy about the case *to us*.[2] We may not be lying or adorning a story, but we are choosing a perspective from which to view a case, and when those choices are made in composing the case study, other possible choices become invisible. There are standard elements that may be almost universally expected in case summaries (such as identifying whether a patient is competent or has decisional capacity, and if not, who the decision maker is and under what governing rule [legal default, HCPA, etc.]), but many aspects of what is noteworthy about a case will be idiosyncratically determined. A person sensitized to issues of faith, gender, culture, or socioeconomic status may focus on or preferentially include these issues, where another person might personally note the presence of such features during the case consultation itself but not center or even mention them in a particular case narrative if they do not play a significant role.

The conclusion I have arrived at after considering "The Zadeh Scenario" and accompanying peer reviews is that if quality attestation is to be largely evaluated based on the case narratives submitted to the judging panel, we must develop a fairly uniform standard for case reports themselves, which is distinct from developing a uniform standard for how a consultation is conducted.[3] In what follows, I note several features of the peer reviews accompanying the Finder case that belie different

[1]For example, consider some of the ways commenters describe Finder's narrative: "wondrously rich;" "polished;" "wonderfully detailed and engaging;" "rich and thoughtful;" a "gift." Though some of this praise is (rightfully) due to gratitude for the fact that Finder makes himself vulnerable in this new mechanism for peer review, it is also an honest assessment of the way in which the narrative is written. Clearly the commenters did not shirk from challenging elements of the narrative due to their praise, but we know from the fields of psychology and sociology that style affects assessment. For example, in the "illusory effect," a message delivered repeatedly is believed more frequently. By repeating claims about "caring for" or "listening to" a patient or family, a consultant could affect an assessment of the case narrative (and thus, the consultation itself) as including evidence that a consultant had the right attitude towards the participants.

[2]As Tod Chambers puts it in his volume about the topic of written cases, *The Fiction of Bioethics*, "What ethicists have generally ignored is that cases – the data by which they test the relevance of moral theory – are fictions. That is, they are made up, constructed and thus follow conventions of representation that *inevitably bias how one understands this information*" (1999, p. 10; emphasis added).

[3]Obviously in this case, Finder and Bliton have not conceived of the volume as focusing on what they argue is a paradigm case narrative. The purpose of the case narrative for the volume and the purpose of case studies written as part of a dossier for quality evaluation may be quite different. Therefore my comments are not directed at this volume's device in particular, but rather, at the more general activity of evaluating consultants and consultations via written reports. (This also raises the question of what to call such writing: "case study" implies a quite distilled summary of a case, while "case narrative" implies a more contextualized account that invites the reader to consider stakeholders more as characters, with personalities, interior lives, and motivations. A discussion of what we should expect from cases summarized for attestation purposes should start with what to call them, and what general tenor they should have within this continuum of possibilities.)

notions of what should be included in a case summary. This may -- or may not -- in turn belie different notions of what questions should be explored as part of doing clinical ethics consultation as a practice.

Disparate Targets of Commentaries

The overall perception a reader of the case and peer reviews is left with is of an impressionistic landscape. Reviewers pick and choose, some working chronologically through the case, others simply picking up pieces they find noteworthy and elaborating on their presence or absence from the case narrative. The organization and focus of each peer review is *sui generis*; they are anything but standardized. While there are a few commonalities, most notably with respect to procedure, the peer reviews diverge quite significantly from each other. Two articles observe that it is not immediately obvious that this *is* a clinical ethics consultation (Tarzian, who concludes after discussion that it is a case consultation, and Rosell & Johnson, who ask but do not explicitly answer this question).

I think this unsystematic approach accurately represents the state of the field. But this must be changed if quality improvement is really what we are after. Systems help to control for the fact of cognitive limitation. We all know healthcare providers should wash their hands, for example, but it took a fairly rigid study and assurance mechanisms to reveal how frequently that did not happen and how controlling for hand-washing and other straightforward, already-verified practices could dramatically affect patient well-being (Haynes et al. 2009). Establishing a system that controls for human cognitive limitations (such as forgetfulness) merely does a better job of making what is desired actually happen than does leaving it up to chance. If case narratives are to be the coin of the new realm of attestation and quality improvement, systematicity in reporting is necessary.[4] Systems establish standards to which individual instances can be compared for adherence; without a system in case reporting, for example, we cannot immediately judge whether a consultation was poor, middling, or excellent based on how the report is written or on what is and is not included. If all we have to evaluate the case is a written report, and we lack a standard for evaluating the written report, we lack a true standard for evaluating a case. And so, questions about method in consultation become, under an attestation model, questions about method in consultation *summaries*. We must articulate the links between what should be done in a consultation and what must be included in a case report.

To illustrate this point, consider two categories of observations represented in Part Two's peer reviews: proceduralism, and feminist and multicultural issues. Not

[4] I recognize that a likely consequence of systematizing or standardizing the case report will be a flattening of richness and detail. But flattening of variation is exactly the point of systems and standards, and it is not clear to me how one might steer between this Scylla and Charybdis. However, it does suggest that case studies or reports for credentialing purposes (in which careers might eventually be at stake) can exist simultaneously with richer narratives meant for other venues.

all peer reviewers mention both; procedural concerns are cited in four of the five peer reviews, cultural concerns by only three, and feminist concerns by only one. Several other concerns are each mentioned by only one peer reviewer. What do these differences tell us about the practice of consultation and about the practice of writing consultation reports?

Proceduralism

By "proceduralism," I mean a focus on proper consultation procedures as evidenced by the case narrative. Tarzian focuses on proceduralism most clearly, as evidenced in her subtitle, "A Focus on Process," and notes that her experience as a chair and member of two different task forces on setting standards in clinical ethics consultation left her with "an appreciation for procedural standards in health care ethics consultation" (Tarzian 2018: 75). Her initial comments, for example, focus on whether this case actually constituted an ethics consultation, and whether it was a *case* consultation or something else; to answer these questions, she turns to the *Core Competencies for Healthcare Ethics Consultation* (ASBH 2011; hereafter "CC"), the current standard in the field, if there is one. Later, she observes that in "The Zadeh Scenario," "there is ambiguity in several procedural aspects of how this consultation was handled," such as whether the role of the former consultant (Moore) was clarified for staff and whether Finder clarified what role he himself would play in the case, with the ultimate question being, Who is really in charge of the case and of communicating with various stakeholders? (Tarzian 2018: 79). Another ambiguity Tarzian comments on is the extent to which medical uncertainty (and the accompanying ethical uncertainty) regarding appropriate treatments was articulated both for health care providers and the patient's family; she points out that "a strategy for determining how these decisions are made" is missing (Tarzian 2018: 83).

Armstrong similarly focuses on procedures by commenting positively on the fact that Finder prepares for the consultation by reviewing the electronic medical record and notifying the attending that he is now involved in the case. However, like Tarzian, Armstrong also wonders whether Finder clarified his role with the family, and why an account of who is making decisions (and why) is missing from the narrative.[5] As practicing CECs will know, there are probably more "informal" or "curbside" consultations than formal ones, and Armstrong points out that "a line can and should be drawn between creating a safe space to discuss and examine moral feelings and a responsibility to follow-up and take action on issues uncovered during such discussions." Because Finder describes both formal and informal requests for consultation, yielding uncertainty about which this case should involve, Armstrong is highlighting the need for the field to create appropriate procedures for these different kinds of consultations.

[5] Armstrong goes further than Tarzian with this concern, offering an extended commentary on "the missing patient" in Finder's narrative.

Hynds' first comment is that consultations should occur "upon request" (that is, not "self-authorize[d]"), so as to avoid the role of the Ethics Police, and observes that it is not clear whether the first consultant in this case (Dr. Moore) was formally consulted. He also wonders about the presumably "hierarchic relationship" between Dr. Finder and Dr. Moore (Hynds 2018: 92) and about the "seemingly unstructured or semi-structured" engagement of consultants with participants (Hynds 2018: 89). He recommends, too, that while Finder explains that consultants in this case met with stakeholders multiple times (and alone), it is better if "interventions are kept to a minimum and all the main players are generally present" (Hynds 2018: 90). The main procedural concerns in Hynds' peer review thus concern the formality and source of the consult request, the appropriate structure of interactions with stakeholders, and the professional relationship between consultants.

Frolic & Rubin, like Tarzian and Armstrong, comment on the apparent lack of role clarity in this case. Not only was the role unclear, they suggest, other procedures were as well. For example, procedural clarity was not evident in this case regarding the "various phases of ethics consultation;" it is not clear from the narrative whether the "ethics consultation in this case contributed to any positive outcome, beyond a good relationship between Finder and the family" (Frolic and Rubin 2018: 59); and it is unclear "if and how the voices of the bedside staff were included in the consultation process" (Frolic and Rubin 2018: 59). Many of these procedural issues are attributed to a lack of "formalization of both the ethics consultant's role and process" (Frolic and Rubin 2018: 59).

Four of the five peer reviewers included procedural concerns in their remarks,[6] but it is noteworthy that they did not all cite the same procedural concerns. The most frequently cited procedural issue was that "The Zadeh Scenario" does not demonstrate that Finder made his role, or that of his colleague Dr. Moore, clear to the patient's family or the medical staff. (It is worth noting, though, that he may have and simply chose not to mention this in the narrative.) Beyond this node of agreement, however, stated concerns about procedure vary. Armstrong mentions the importance of distinguishing between formal and informal consultations; Hynds stresses the importance that consultants should wait to be called (rather than being proactive) and that consultation meetings should usually involve all stakeholders; and Frolic & Rubin observe that a lack of formalization of the process of consultation may be causing a number of problems.

The peer reviews are not mutually incompatible, so I do not mean to suggest that they demonstrate some radical disagreement about clinical ethics consultation. But they do present quite different pictures of what a case narrative should include. This

[6] I have not included in this count Rosell & Johnson, who describe their commentary as a phenomenological analysis in an "interrogative" mode and do not couch their comments in "procedural" terms. However, many of their remarks may have procedural elements – for example, they note that patients have the right not to receive particular treatments or care from particular providers, and that they have the right under law and because of respect for autonomy to make decisions for themselves.

may help explain the focus on procedure, because it is an area where we might hope for some consensus. However, even in the comments on procedural issues, these peer reviews reveal different priorities.

Multicultural and Feminist Perspectives

A quote from Dr. Moore indicates that the family is Persian, and three of the peer reviewers take up this fact for discussion. Rosell & Johnson observe only in passing that "the narrative gives several indicators of cultural normative difference in regard to making end of life decisions" (Rosell and Johnson 2018: 103), while Tarzian and Armstrong offer more extended comments. Tarzian raises the idea of "cultural competence" in providing health care, and asserts that "[i]t's clear that this [cultural difference] contributed substantially to the perceived conflicts between the Hamadani family and the staff caring for Mrs. Hamadani" (Tarzian 2018: 78). However, she notes that although Finder recognized these possible cultural issues in the case, "it's unclear whether or how he addressed these conflicts in his role as the ethics consultant" (Tarzian 2018: 80). Armstrong challenges whether we should assume, based on the family's Persian culture, that the patient would have wanted her family to make decisions for her.

Encountering a patient and family with a cultural foundation that might affect their approach to decision-making is common in clinical ethics consultation. Cultural difference can be a linchpin for an entire case – or completely irrelevant. Here, two out of five peer reviews did not even include mention of the issue; but even of the three that did, the responses to the cultural element of the case have next to no overlap. To be specific, one flags it but does not assess Dr. Finder's performance or narrative based on it; one assumes that the cultural issue "contributed substantially to the perceived conflicts" and faults Finder for not discussing how he incorporated these concerns into his consultation; and one notes that culture is not dispositive of wishes when a patient has not stated her own wishes.

Gender and social norms can also play a significant role in clinical ethics cases, but only one author, Armstrong, comments on the role of gender in the case at hand. This case involves an incapacitated mother with one son and two daughters, but the only apparent candidate for decision-maker appears to be the son. Armstrong observes that the daughters have only first names but the son has a first and last name (and is called "Mr. Zadeh" in the narrative), and that "none of the female characters' opinions regarding treatment independent of Mr. Zadeh's interpretation are explored…both the patient and her daughters form a silent chorus for Mr. Zadeh" (Armstrong 2018: 69). It is worth noting that only one of the five peer reviewers found the issue of gender worth noting.

Other Issues

In addition to procedural and cultural concerns, several other concerns are mentioned in Part Two, though in most cases only one author mentions each feature. Armstrong, Rosell & Johnson, and Frolic & Rubin all focus on the absence of the patient's voice in "The Zadeh Scenario," but mostly in passing. Rosell & Johnson remark that "Mrs. Hamadani is mostly absent in this consultation activity" (Rosell and Johnson 2018: 106); Frolic & Rubin raise the question about what the patient wants as the final and most important category in a list of questions that are not answered in the narrative; Armstrong, in her discussion of "the missing patient," notes that by not mentioning any conversation with the patient about her wishes, "the case appears to presume that she did not wish to be involved in decision-making, or that her wishes were adequately represented by her children" (Armstrong 2018: 68).

Armstrong and Frolic & Rubin comment on Finder's use of the electronic medical record to track readmitted patients who have had ethical issues during past admissions. Frolic & Rubin "worry this could lead to some inadvertent role confusion (what exactly is the ethics consultant contributing by 'checking in' on a previous case?) as well as potential violation of the patient's privacy" (Frolic and Rubin 2018: 58). Armstrong also mentions privacy, but emphasizes more that this practice makes it difficult to know when a consultation has ended, and whether follow-up in this way is part of continuity of care.

Frolic & Rubin also stress the importance of a consultant's self-examination and reflecting critically on one's own practices, noting that Finder does not engage in this practice in this narrative. Armstrong comments that there was evidence of moral distress among healthcare providers, but that Finder does not indicate that this issue was explored at all in the narrative.

Reflections

The peer reviews in Part Two, like "The Zadeh Scenario," are rich, thoughtful, and appropriate. But even if all of them are correct, I cannot help but conclude that no case narrative short of a novella could hope to satisfy all of these informational demands, and perhaps not even then. This is not a judgment about the authors of the case or peer reviews, who are attuned to the limits of this format. They also did not compose their comments on the premise that they were working towards some paradigm in case narrative. This book is not meant to recommend a model for adoption in case studies. However, because Finder's case is (as the peer reviewers note) a much richer, more contextual and detailed narrative than is customary, and yet *still* all five authors in Part Two find much lacking in the description, the conclusions drawn must also hold for case studies in general given that they tend to be much shorter, more generic, and lacking in detail and context. The case study is a limited vehicle, in other words, and if it is to form the basis of attestation in clinical ethics consultation, we must standardize what we expect to see in a case narrative.

Imagine if the peer reviewers on this case comprised an attestation panel. Although there is some overlap in their positive comments (e.g., most praised Finder for the care he showed the family), there is hardly any overlap in their critical comments. What would this mean for an attestation evaluation of Finder? This returns us to the difference between assessing a consultant's practice and assessing a case report, because the assumption in the attestation model is that the practice can be evaluated via the case report. This assumption is problematic.

First, if these peer reviews are any indication, authors will have idiosyncratic framing mechanisms for writing case reports, and evaluators will have idiosyncratic responses to cases. For example, Finder may have noticed, explored, and eliminated a feminist concern from the narrative because it played no role, and only one commenter (Armstrong) mentions feminist concerns in her paper. The lack of mention of feminist concerns in the case is merely absence of evidence, not evidence of absence. Armstrong's concern with the way the case narrative is written (e.g., that the daughters have only first names and the son a first and last name) may be legitimate, but it may be a concern with Finder's *narrative choices*, not a concern with his consultation practice (except by tenuous inference between narrative choices and consultation practices).

Three peer reviewers mention cultural issues, reacting to Dr. Moore's statement that the family is Persian and to Finder's conclusion that "cultural elements" may have played a role in the case. But there are many more possible interpretations of this case narrative. We have no actual evidence that *culture* was at play, rather than religion, family dynamics, economic issues, etc. The fact that the family is Persian (are the children also Persian? Or are they Persians born in the US?) ends up being an easy heuristic for "value difference," but it is a heuristic that may mislead. It is not implausible that culture affected the case, but culture is not monolithic, and we characterize individuals inappropriately if we assume that individual beliefs follow directly from cultural context. Finder may have been blind to these issues, exquisitely attuned to them, or somewhere in between; the commenters may have chosen to focus on "pet" concerns, may have drilled right to the heart of the case, or somewhere in between. We simply lack the information we would need to establish which is the case.

In the account of the proposed Attestation model (Kodish et al. 2013), the authors recognize the problem of interrater reliability (which is part, but not all, of the problem outlined above) and offer a mechanism to address it. As the evaluation of the portfolios moved forward, the 12 members of the assessment group "convened to establish assessment metrics" based on the portfolios they had received, then piloted the instruments for face validity and construct validity. It is the problem of "construct validity" – "the ability of the test to measure what is intended" – that I mean to focus on. What I have been illustrating in discussing these case commentaries is the problem of our lack of standards in case reports. If we think it is important to include in a case report a discussion of even those issues that played no significant role during the case, we must offer a template or framework of case reports that prompts discussion of such issues, even if that amounts to a statement that this issue was not relevant to the case.[7]

Conclusion

Quality improvement procedures only work if they capture all and only what is appropriate to the task. We have a double-layer problem in the idea of an attestation model of assessing clinical ethics consultation, because we lack standards at the level of the individual consultation, and we haven't even begun to discuss standard expectations of case summaries. This model of an extended case study with commentaries is worth repeating as we develop standards in the field, because such a process generates the diverse elements of a consultation and its reporting that practitioners find important.[8] As the field's assessment mechanisms are shaped, these elements must be standardized and promulgated so that authors of case reports know the bases on which their cases will be assessed. Without clear direction regarding the necessary elements in a case report, attestation of abilities based on case summaries will be impossible, unfair, or arbitrary.

References

Armstrong K (2018) Telling about engagement is not enough: seeking the "ethics" of ethics consultation in clinical ethics case reports. In: Finder SG, Bliton MJ (eds) Peer review, peer education, and modeling in the practice of clinical ethics consultation: the Zadeh project. Springer, Cham, pp 63–73

Chambers T (1999) The fiction of bioethics: cases as literary texts. Routledge, New York

Finder SG (2018) The Zadeh scenario. In: Finder SG, Bliton MJ (eds) Peer review, peer education, and modeling in the practice of clinical ethics consultation: the Zadeh project. Springer, Cham, pp 21–42

Frolic A, Rubin SB (2018) Critical self-reflection as moral practice: a collaborative meditation on peer review in ethics consultation. In: Finder SG, Bliton MJ (eds) Peer review, peer education, and modeling in the practice of clinical ethics consultation: the Zadeh project. Springer, Cham, pp 47–61

Haynes AB, Weiser TG, Berry WR, for the safe surgery saves lives study group et al (2009) A surgical safety checklist to reduce morbidity and mortality in global population. NEJM 360:491–449

[7] One possibility for ensuring comprehensiveness both during a consultation and in a case report is the use of a standardized checklist. I gave a presentation on such a mechanism at the International Conference on Clinical Ethics Consultation 2015, in New York, NY.

[8] For example, journals could add a regular feature emulating this approach, and conferences such as the American Society for Bioethics and Humanities (ASBH) and the International Conference for Clinical Ethics consultation could provide conference slots for panels arranged for this commentary.

Hynds J (2018) Ethics consultation, professional praxis, and what it means to be a "consultant". In: Finder SG, Bliton MJ (eds) Peer review, peer education, and modeling in the practice of clinical ethics consultation: the Zadeh project. Springer, Cham, pp 85–97

Kodish E, Fins JJ, Braddock C et al (2013) Quality attestation for clinical ethics consultants: a two-step model from the American Society for Bioethics and Humanities. Hastings Cent Rep 43(5):26–36

Rosell T, Johnson B (2018) This may, or may not, be an ethics consultation. In: Finder SG, Bliton MJ (eds) Peer review, peer education, and modeling in the practice of clinical ethics consultation: the Zadeh project. Springer, Cham, pp 99–107

Tarzian AJ (2018) Ethics consultation for Mrs. Hamadani: a focus on process. In: Finder SG, Bliton MJ (eds) Peer review, peer education, and modeling in the practice of clinical ethics consultation: the Zadeh project. Springer, Cham, pp 75–84

PART FOUR
CRITICAL INQUIRY INTO PARTS ONE, TWO, AND THREE (ON THE WAY TOWARDS PEER REVIEW)

Brief Summary of the Essays in Part Four

Part Four brings into focus several additional matters that must be addressed in any format for peer review and evaluation of clinical ethics consultation. Even more so than the preceding Parts, summarizing these essays does insufficient justice to the maturity and intelligence of the insights expressed in their carefully developed perspectives. These contributions convey the authors' reading of the previous essays, their proposals for methods and criteria for evaluation, the implications for ethics consultants and consultation practices, and the need to engage the multiple discourses in the field. Not only do these perspectives sharpen the concerns evident in the preceding chapters, they highlight the significant challenges for any ethics consultant about his or her own experiences and practice. Taken together, these chapters display the challenges that must be answered by those evaluating ethics consultation and entailed activities, especially when evaluations are conducted from a context, time, and place different than those in which the consultation was conducted – with perhaps different conceptions about the underlying commitments that support ethics consultation.

Stella Reiter-Theil and Jan Schürmann begin with "Evaluating Clinical Ethics Support: On What Grounds Do We Make Judgments About Reports of Ethics Consultation?" In addition to clearly identifying the need to recognize the conceptual and practical significance of internal as well as external standards for evaluation, Reiter-Theil and Schürmann raise another crucial topic to consider. They ask this sort of question: If we lack presentation of the phenomenological, interpretive, and existential elements that contribute to the normative understanding for a particular situation, to what extent can we legitimately identify, assess, and make some appraisal about the analytical and interventional elements for ethics consultations? By way of response, they include in their outline of criteria to use for evaluation the idea that "criteria regarding the doing of ethics consultation may require different kinds of material evidence than the criteria regarding the documentation of ethics consultation" (Reiter-Theil and Schürmann 2018: 174). They further describe an integrative model that attempts to balance these various elements by suggesting that these represent what they call a "repertoire" of relevant activities and approaches. Keeping that in mind, they go on to suggest that it is important for those being reviewed and those doing the review "to agree in advance about the internal as well as the external standards that are to be utilized in evaluation" (Reiter-Theil and Schürmann 2018: 176).

Any such agreement, as Jeff Bishop proposes in "Doing Well or Doing Good in Ethics Consultation," would be better served by recognizing that, as a clinical activity, "clinical ethics consultation is a kind of doing that is a local form of moral enquiry, seeking not just to achieve medical – or clinical ethical – goals, but to enact human goods" (Bishop 2018: 181). In support of this proposal, Bishop critically examines the philosophical tenets typically used to underwrite the methods outlined by Bruce and Aulisio, making his argument that "proceduralism is at the heart of all four methodologies" presented by Bruce. Bishop then engages the explication of rules by Agich to clearly remind ethics consultants and peer reviewers that rules translated and standardized into guidelines are abstractions that "become the codes, procedures, and policies to now be applied by ethicists to all cases" (Bishop 2018: 183). He agrees with Agich that making these translations in order to traverse among clinical and organizational levels of activities and assessment, for instance those presented by Reiter-Theil and Schürmann, requires a great deal of caution and care. One primary ingredient of such care that Bishop reflects is gained from insights that phenomenology brings to clinical ethics because what "phenomenology asks us to do is to bracket our preconceptions – even our procedural preconceptions – about what we think matters in a case, and to attend to the things that matter to the patient, to the patient's family, and to the patient's caregivers" (Bishop 2018: 187). "In fact," Bishop goes on to say, "'The Zadeh Scenario' is a narrative of what matters to the patient and the family. This narrative is a narrative describing the bringing forth of goods possible in dying. With this narrative, Finder challenges us to bracket our procedures and policies and guidelines" (Bishop 2018: 189).

Guy Widdershoven, Bert Molewijk, and Suzanne Metselaar bring this section to a close with a sensitive and careful elaboration that clarifies several core elements for peer review. Their essay, "Peer Review and Beyond: Towards a Dialogical Approach of Quality in Ethics Support," probes several ideas about the contents that elements in a story should portray in order to serve as a part of a peer review. They clarify and discuss a central theme of the book, specifically, the differences in assessments that can, and will, occur among different peer reviewers. In response, they highlight several elements which, although complex, should be included. First, there are elements, orientations actually, they call "the attention for details" and "the sensitivity for how facts in the case (e.g. behavior, words used, medical situation) are interpreted" (Widdershoven et al. 2018: 195). A second element considers the story of the ethics consultation under review to suggest that these stories "should focus on the identification of ethical elements of a clinical situation, the analysis of values and norms of the stakeholders involved in that clinical situation, and the way in which value conflicts are made explicit and turned into an issue for deliberation" (Widdershoven et al. 2018: 197). They also make explicit a major theme threaded throughout the book, saying, "it is the dialogue between interpretations that holds out the promise for actual growth in understanding what the quality of clinical ethics practice entails" (Widdershoven et al. 2018: 198). Their proposal is that such elements then can be exemplified through additional interactions to stimulate "com parison and learning to see the case better by sharing commonalities and differences," and in that way bring this sort of dialogue into what they call a "responsive evaluation" (Widdershoven et al. 2018: 201) among perspectives held within a broader and more inclusive group of stakeholders in a healthcare environment to enable a more extensive interaction with the moral circumstances and commitments under consideration.

Evaluating Clinical Ethics Support: On What Grounds Do We Make Judgments About Reports of Ethics Consultation?

Stella Reiter-Theil and Jan Schürmann

Introduction

In this chapter, we explore the question of on what grounds reports of clinical ethics support in general, including especially clinical ethics consultation, can or should be evaluated when using a peer review system, and we propose five core points to consider. It is our contention that to evaluate clinical ethics consultation within a peer review system aiming at transparency and fairness, one has to rely on defined and shared criteria of evaluation, i.e. an evaluation standard (although the term "standard" is by no means trivial, this chapter will not focus on its thorough clarification). Such a standard is grounded on a (defined and shared) conceptualization of how an ethics consultation should be performed. Obviously, there are different ways of doing clinical ethics consultation also corresponding with different evaluation standards (Pfaefflin et al. 2009; Schürmann et al. 2013). When evaluating a performed ethics consultation (according to a given documentation), we can roughly distinguish between an internal standard, which refers to the conceptualization of clinical ethics consultation held by the respective consultant or by the assessed clinical ethics support service (CESS) themselves, and external standards. Most important is the way *how* an external standard is being defined: Is it just the standard of another service or colleague? Or is it the result of a larger consensus-building process of a relevant body representing a larger group of colleagues such as the guidelines of the ASBH (2011)? Or does it even rely on the "evidence" of related research? An external standard, however, may rest on criteria that are not – or not fully – accepted by the evaluated CESS or individual ethics consultant. However, identifying the internal standard of an observed ethics consultant's work may also be

S. Reiter-Theil (✉) · J. Schürmann
Department of Clinical Ethics, University Hospital Basel / University of Basel, Basel, Switzerland
e-mail: s.reiter-theil@unibas.ch; jan.schuermann@unibas.ch

S. G. Finder, M. J. Bliton (eds.), *Peer Review, Peer Education, and Modeling in the Practice of Clinical Ethics Consultation: The Zadeh Project*,
https://doi.org/10.1007/978-3-319-90955-4_12

challenging: Has it been published, and does it still apply to the recent case at hand? Is it clear or may there be misinterpretations? From the evaluator's perspective the responsibility for making an internal standard known and unequivocal lies with the "author" of the material. The potential gap between internal and external standards marks a methodological difficulty that as such has to be addressed within peer review evaluation.

Summarizing, we suggest that clinical ethics consultation should be evaluated by an internal standard held to be relevant by the respective consultant or CESS; moreover, we think that this internal standard must be in accordance with a general framework for the specific ethics consultation to be accessible to peer review evaluation. As a consequence of this coupled approach, the process of evaluation will avoid getting lost in a merely subjective, self-referential circle.

Besides different standards, there are also different kinds of methodological approaches to evaluate performed clinical ethics consultations, e.g. embedded research (Reiter-Theil 2012; Reiter-Theil and Schürmann 2016), analysis of (oral or written) reports, or analysis of videos. In analyzing oral or written reports, one can rely on different types of material such as case vignettes, records, narratives or feedback. Each type has different merits leading to specific strengths and weaknesses regarding the assessment, the data and conclusions. We suggest that an analysis relying on a combined report, including narrative and record, might best account for the weaknesses of each approach.

Finder's "The Zadeh Scenario" offers a rich narrative and in our eyes seems to implicitly communicate his internal standard of how to do clinical ethics consultation. He has, more importantly, made explicit his approach elsewhere – it may be described as a phenomenological-hermeneutical approach (Bliton and Finder 1999). In the first-level peer reviews given in this volume, the peer reviewers do not seem to embrace this approach in its full extension, as they assess Finder's narrative in "The Zadeh Scenario" using an approach that Bruce describes appropriately as "proceduralism" (Bruce 2018) – an approach that we consider, in this case, to be an external standard.

The type of report Finder has provided – a written narrative – is, according to our understanding, suitable to assess conversational, phenomenological, hermeneutical and existentialistic aspects of an ethics consultation. We think that Finder's narrative does well in addressing these aspects, with some shortcomings regarding the hermeneutical criterion. Considering further criteria of the proposed framework – analytical, normative, interventional – "The Zadeh Scenario" falls short in providing the reader with a more comprehensive report and, especially, reflection.

Critical Appraisal of the Commentaries

Interestingly, each of the second-level commentaries (Part Three) achieve different things. Accordingly, in order to clarify their particular objectives, each must be addressed individually.

Bruce

Bruce explores the methods referred to by the first-level reviewers to assess Finder's performance. Under "method" Bruce understands the systematic procedure, technique, or mode of inquiry employed during ethics consultation. Bruce presents four main methods discussed in clinical ethics literature: principlism, casuistry, narrative ethics, and clinical pragmatism. While the peer reviewers hardly refer to principlism and casuistry, they invoke several aspects of narrative ethics and clinical pragmatism. Regarding narrative ethics they refer to criteria such as engagement in dialogue, usage of open and well-crafted questions, involvement of all individuals concerned, or the richness of the story. Regarding clinical pragmatism, they refer to several procedural criteria: identifying the main ethical concern (of the requestor), clarifying the role of the ethics consultant, identifying and justifying appropriate treatment options, appealing to professional, legal or ethical standards, focusing on problem-solving, etc.

Bruce suggests that in using both narrative and procedural criteria the reviewers implicitly point to a new method which she calls "proceduralism." According to this approach, clinical ethics consultation should follow a systematic procedure that refers to the cited procedural criteria. It includes, however, as an additional procedural step any activities referring to the narrative criteria mentioned above. This, she argues, enables proceduralism to include the benefits of narrative ethics – discovery of meanings and values, context/case sensitivity, empathic support – and yet be effectively oriented at solving the ethical problem. Moreover it yields a distinct standard of procedural justification in ethics consultation: "Proceduralism allows for internal consistency and justificatory force to the extent that certain steps should be followed and justifications provided if these steps are not followed" (Bruce 2018: 123).

Bruce ends with four preliminary recommendations for clinical ethicists who get their ethics consultation assessed by peer review: (1) be explicit in your approach and justify deviations, (2) identify the nature of the ethical concern, (3) be explicit in your role, (4) identify and justify which interventions are considered inappropriate.

We tend to agree with Bruce's reconstruction of the method used by the first-level peer reviewers. However, it has to be acknowledged that proceduralism is an external standard that seems to deviate considerably from the internal standard used by Finder. Also, the reviewers' methodological conformity appears coincidental as several studies did indeed show the prevalence of principlism as method of ethics consultation (e.g. Slowther et al. 2012: 212). It would, thus, be at least somewhat premature to recommend the criteria of proceduralism as a kind of gold standard for peer review assessment.

Regarding Bruce's preliminary recommendations for reviewed clinical ethicists, it's not entirely clear whether these are meant to be "recommendations" referring to the *doing* of ethics consultation or referring to its *documentation*. As Rasmussen makes perfectly clear, these standards have to be distinguished and their relationship has to be clarified. We think that these recommendations capture important features that any kind of (oral or written) report has to display in order to be suited for peer review assessment.

Aulisio

The case narrative itself, rather than the first-level peer reviews, is further appreciated by Aulisio who raises a number of most interesting questions, e.g. on the role of the ethics consultant, the significance of autonomy- versus community-centric value sets, on hearing the voice of the patient, on the way of taking over a case from a colleague, on the request of a patient's family, to mention just a selection. Aulisio presents, instead of answering these questions, three "meta-methodological" lessons for method in clinical ethics consultation. They are as follows:

1. *Identifying and analyzing the underlying value conflict or uncertainties*

For Aulisio, the family's perception that they hold the value of "respecting and caring for parents" while suggesting that this was not the case in the surrounding majority U.S. culture, needs to be further explored so as to gain a broader understanding of the meaning of "respecting and caring for parents" as he – convincingly – supposes that the prevailing divergence might lie in the respective interpretations. Does "respecting and caring for parents" mean clinging to maximum life-supporting treatment, even given the evidence of burdening the patient with marginal expected benefit? Or could "respecting and caring for parents" also be understood as engaging in the search for the authentic wishes and needs of the patient, even if those may contradict the family's traditional customs or beliefs?

In his commentary (discussion of which is below), Agich criticizes Finder's approach when performing the ethics consultation arguing that he acted more like a "sensitive communicator and counselor for [the] family" (Agich 2018: 147). However, even in that role, one of the primary tasks would have been to clarify the values and commitments that were at stake in different possible interpretations. Aulisio's impression is that the expected value clarification did not take place (or was at least not provided in the narrative). Thus, rather than suggesting that Finder simply took on the role of another profession, the question must be asked, why did he act as he did, and on what grounds? More specifically, the question here is whether Finder's phenomenological framework of doing ethics consultation actually contributes to – or at least permits – a better understanding of the values and commitments (along with real or perceived conflicts and uncertainty) at stake?

2. *Clarifying who has the decision making authority*

Aulisio is quite adamant that all healthcare professionals, including ethics consultants, should maintain (or establish) respect for the authority of the patient in decision-making. He thus identifies as a "mistake" that the locus of decision-making appears to have been placed upon Mrs. Hamadani's family (instead of Mrs.

Hamadani herself). Although this may be an unusually strong expression – in the sense that the talk of "mistakes" is still somewhat uncommon in clinical ethics literature (Rubin and Zoloft 2000) – it is the case that many nations (including our own home countries, Germany and Switzerland) have laws that reinforce ethical standards according to which, when patients lack capacity to participate in decision-making, healthcare professionals not ask patients' relatives or legal representatives for their own preferences regarding patient care; instead, they should be asked about the patient's values and preferences. Whatever else it is the role entails, therefore, it is an ethics consultant's task to ensure that this norm is followed. Against this frame, Aulisio also outlines a key role of the care team: to articulate the range of medically acceptable options and to offer clear recommendations. This includes, we would add, the task of articulating the limitations of interventions that do not make sense or create (moral) trouble such as the experience of practicing substandard pain control or futile care.

3. *Taking care that the patient's voice is being heard*

This serious concern of Aulisio's is illustrated by a label that is most telling: the "secondary patient." He warns us to prevent making "secondary patients" of family members with the risk of not only shifting the locus of decision-making but also the focus of care to the relatives rather than focusing on the patient. In explaining this challenge, Aulisio acknowledges the importance of nonetheless paying attention to the needs of the troubled family and making available relevant support from other appropriate professionals or resource groups. However, the question must be raised whether any limits or exceptions to the rule could be claimed from a moral perspective when the needs of a "secondary" patient (family member) have to be prioritized. For example, if a husband who promised to take care of his terminally ill, hospitalized wife is overburdened by this task and gets ill himself, his needs, as the "secondary patient," may indeed have to be prioritized over the wishes of the primary patient. This can be justified by the bridge principle "ought implies can": after falling ill, the husband has reached his limits and cannot maintain his promise to take care of his wife, and as a result, two primary patients emerge who both have needs and rights in themselves, even when they fall short of reciprocal wish-fulfilling.

We suppose that in Finder's case another option should be considered: some family members may have become a "primary patient" in their own right even if this is not explicitly communicated. According to "The Zadeh Scenario," this has not been an issue in the case. There is, however, another significant question: are there good reasons to suggest that Finder might have perceived such a critical situation within the Hamadani family? Did he perceive – without articulating – that some family members were in some kind of critical need situation where their "salvation," their moral or mental stability, required prioritized understanding or support because they otherwise might not have been able to escape "guilt" by consenting to palliative care goals?

On the whole, Aulisio's commentary is not only insightful and well supported by references, but also refreshing in his explicit questioning and constructive criticism.

It is also appreciated that he explicitly addresses how an ethics consultant is dealing with the normative dimension of a case – and the related tasks in the role of being an ethics consultant. Aulisio doesn't further elaborate on the status of his "meta-methodological" rules, apart from saying that they "are at a level of generality that makes them […] compatible with and relevant for a wide variety of more specific models, approaches and methods of doing ethics consultation in health care settings" (Aulisio 2018: 128). We may account for this status by saying that these rules belong to a general framework describing what it means to do ethics consultation in the clinical context – a framework that is mandatory for peer review assessment of ethics consultation. Justifying such a status, however, cannot be done merely by exemplary case analysis, but requires conceptual analysis of both clinical and social norms as well as a robust consensus-building process among clinical ethics consultants.

Agich

In the first part of his chapter, Agich clarifies his understanding of doing clinical ethics consultation. In short, he understands ethics consultation essentially as a "reflective practice" in which the ethics consultant reflectively and responsibly engages in specific actions and communications such as gathering information, assessment, interpretation, planning meetings, analysis or providing advice. In doing so, the ethics consultant contributes to a hermeneutical process of giving meaning to the circumstances of the clinical case. This process builds on the conceptual, factual, evaluative and ethical views of the patient, family, and health care professionals involved, but also depends on a wider framework of social meanings. Agich considers three methodological implications of his reflective practice approach: (1) in order to define the distinctive set of rules guiding an ethics consultation, we have to neutrally describe the essential features of the doings in the practice of clinical ethics itself – and not, for instance, refer to ethical theory or methods; (2) the ability to enact these rules in practice is learned by way of actually performing and experiencing clinical ethics consultation – and not by studying formal codes, procedures, or guidelines; (3) in order to review an ethics consultation, we have to construe the whole "history" of that ethics consultation – not just look at its outcome. The history is ideally a set of critical reflections on all aspects of an ethics consultation which may be manifest in different kinds of reports (records, written or spoken narratives etc.).

In the second part, Agich focuses on four procedural features of Finder's performance: direct communication among ethics consultation team members, written ethics consultation records, the role of the ethics consultants, and the dynamic character of clinical ethics consultations. According to Agich, the direct communication between Finder and Moore was effective (which is essential). Similarly, Agich acknowledges the importance of having written records in the course of ethics consultation. In terms of the role of Finder, Agich is a bit more critical, briefly discussing that it seems to have been more that of a "sensitive communicator and counselor for [the] family" (Agich 2018: 147) than of an ethics consultant. As regards the dynamic character of clinical ethics consultation, Agich is again more positive, noting that this feature is admirably displayed by "The Zadeh Scenario." In the end, however, Agich questions the adequacy of Finder's narrative as a learning model for dealing with the normative dimension in ethics consultation.

In describing his reflective practice approach of clinical ethics consultation, Agich provides, according to our terminology, an external standard for evaluating Finder's ethics consultation. However, it remains unclear whether this evaluation standard is the same as the standard used by Finder or the first-level reviewers. We suppose that Agich's approach actually is quite similar to Finder's in its emphasis on engagement in a hermeneutical process with the individuals involved in a clinical case (for a description of Finder's approach, see our Discussion below). It lacks, in other words, a focus on referring to an explicit procedural framework – a statement that is paramount for the peer reviewers, as Bruce points out. Thus, in contrast to the first-level reviewers, Agich refers to an external standard that may count as internal as well. But this is only coincidental – we argue that for proper peer review assessment both internal and external standards, as well as their relationship, have to be articulated explicitly.

Agich's main criticism of "The Zadeh Scenario" is that it omits critical reflection of normative aspects of the case. This criticism is based on Agich's understanding of ethics consultation as a practice that primarily aims to provide thoughtful advice on *ethical* concerns rather than to provide emotional support for the patient's family. However, it remains unclear in what specific way Finder's performance misses the normative dimension, as Agich does not clarify how ethical concerns should be dealt with according to his own approach. In order to assess the handling of ethical concerns in the practice of clinical ethics by means of peer review assessment, examinee and reviewer have to agree on specific normative evaluation criteria.

The methodological implications Agich mentions also bear on peer review assessment. First, his insistence on the practical embeddedness of the rules guiding clinical ethics consultation reminds us that the evaluation criteria used in peer review have to be specified in view of the actual doings in ethics consultation. Second, in order to assess the whole "history" of clinical ethics consultation, we may have to rely on different kinds of material – not only narratives as in this case.

Rasmussen

Rasmussen's commentary starts by stating a number of limitations that arise for evaluation of ethics consultation when that evaluation is conducted by looking through the lens of the case narrative. Anticipating her clear, concise and constructive conclusion (we will come back to it in the Discussion), this recognition of such limitations reinforces the key message that the evaluation of ethics consultation requires standardization including a uniform standard for case reports themselves – which as she clarifies is distinct from a uniform standard for how a consultation is conducted.

As a kind of illustrative reason for the request for standardization, she explores the diversity of the five first-level peer reviewers in Part Two, with their "disparate targets" and nearly completely different ways of commenting on the case report, the result of which is "few commonalities, most notably with respect to procedure" (Rasmussen 2018: 153). One very basic divergence concerns the question raised in two out of the five peer reviews, namely whether "this *is* a clinical ethics consultation"; only one of the two confirms that this is the case.

In our view, possible triggers for this line of questioning are as follows:

(a) Finder's activity is different from an ethics consultation taking place "on demand", but appears (after the initial demand) to become increasingly self-triggered or -steered over time;
(b) it does not seem to focus on the needs of staff and it is not reported how ethical content matters are processed to the staff's benefit;
(c) although clinical ethics consultation can take place as a response to patient or family request, this does not seem to be the case here: rather, the family was simply asking Finder, in his administrative role as "Director," to remove the first ethics consultant;
(d) if an ethics consultation request is initiated from a staff need, but then shifts to focus on the needs and values of patient or family, some indication of the appropriateness of that shift is needed and must be included in the ethics consultation documentation; and finally,
(e) there seems to be a similarity between the at least partly non-requested involvement of the ethics consultant and the discussed risk of medical over-treatment.

What Rasmussen concludes (correctly, we believe) is that "this unsystematic approach accurately represents the state of the field" and "if case narratives are to be the coin of the new realm of attestation and quality improvement, systematicity in reporting is necessary" (Rasmussen 2018: 153). For further illustration, she picks two categories of observations: proceduralism and then feminist and multicultural issues.

With respect to proceduralism, Rasmussen notes that the authors in Part Two raise various procedural aspects of clinical ethics practice. There is, however, minimal overlap regarding questions about the (clarification of the) ethics consultant's role, similar to what we have discussed in the previous paragraphs in reference to Bruce, Aulisio, and Agich. Regarding feminism and multicultural issues, Rasmussen similarly states that the few responses to cultural elements (by three of the authors) "have next to no overlap" (Rasmussen 2018: 156). More importantly, however, Rasmussen explicitly draws attention to the fact that Armstrong seems to argue (Armstrong 2018: 69) that we should not assume that the patient would have wanted her family to make decisions for her because she is Persian (Rasmussen 2018: 156). Moreover, Rasmussen notes that Armstrong is also the only author who comments on a gender issue, observing that in "The Zadeh Scenario," Finder is calling the two daughters by their first names while calling their brother by his last name (as he does for the patient, always, and only, using "Mrs. Hamadani"). This observation is extended to stating that none of the female characters' opinions were explored. Interestingly, Aulisio did adjust this asymmetry by calling all three children of Mrs. Hamadani by their first names, including Samir, the son. However, this egalitarian approach did not extend to the healthcare (ethics) professionals who kept their last names throughout "The Zadeh Scenario" and the commentaries.

From an intercultural perspective we can point out a difference to some Anglo-American practices. In a continental European culture, a non-reciprocal use of names would be most uncommon among adults (equals) and any deviation would be registered as surprising, especially in a professional context such as a hospital. A distinction exists in most European languages between addressing a person on familiar terms or in the formal form of address by using the personal pronouns of "Du" or "Sie", and it is a common practice, if not a social norm of good style, to respect mutuality (except for relations between, e.g., teachers and children). Thus, these observations seem to indicate that sensitive issues exist not only with regard to gender and communication, but also regarding the representative symbols of professional hierarchy towards patients and relatives.

In her reflections, Rasmussen articulates reservation about the assumption that clinical ethics practice could be evaluated by evaluating the retrospective case report – given the diversity of such reports. This leads to her conclusions that we are facing a double-layer problem: (1) a lack of standards regarding the individual ethics consultation and (2) the lack of standards regarding the ways they are documented. To adequately address these problems, Rasmussen suggests, requires not only standardizing the assessed elements of clinical ethics consultation as well as of clinical ethics consultation reports, but also promulgating these standards among all the participants of the assessment – otherwise, she says, peer review assessment will be "impossible, unfair, or arbitrary" (Rasmussen 2018: 159).

Discussion

The task to reflect methodologically on the peer reviews presented by the authors in Part Two is interpreted differently by each of the four authors in Part Three. This may not come as a surprise, as the concepts of method present a great deal of variety both in terms of theory and practice of clinical ethics consultation. Perhaps due to the difference in objective, there are hardly any open discrepancies between the commentaries in Part Three. One such discrepancy is the different emphasis Bruce and Rasmussen pursue when assessing the conformity among the Part Two reviews. Whereas Bruce suggests that they are similar enough to subsume them under the method of proceduralism, Rasmussen thinks that they hardly share the most basic assumptions – apart from the focus on procedure.

As to the task for Part Four, we acknowledge that each of the previous sets of reflections (Parts Two and Three) provides an opportunity to develop important conclusions about peer review assessment of clinical ethics consultation reports. We summarize these conclusions as follows. In peer review assessment of ethics consultation, (1) internal and external evaluation standards have to be articulated

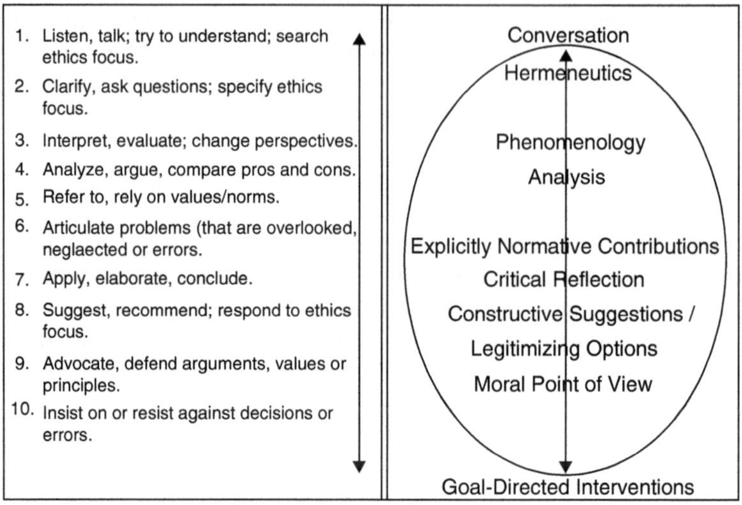

Fig. 1 Inventory and escalating model of dealing with the normative dimension in ethics consultation – the repertoire of an ethics consultant (Reiter-Theil (2009) with friendly permission by Cambridge University Press)

explicitly; (2) reviewee and reviewer have to agree on specific evaluation criteria applying to the actual doings in clinical ethics consultation; (3) these evaluation criteria should conform to a general evaluative framework; (4) that framework has to be validated in a consensus-building process among ethics consultants; (5) evaluation criteria are needed both for the *doing* of ethics consultation and for the *documentation* of ethics consultation; (6) the criteria regarding the doing of ethics consultation may require different kinds of material evidence than the criteria regarding the documentation of ethics consultation.

We rely on an integrative model (Reiter-Theil 2009) as a way of appreciating these suggestions and as a response to the demanding task to locate the divergent criteria of clinical ethics consultation that have emerged from the tableau of opinions into a conceptual framework. This model suggests a repertoire covering activities and approaches to be found in clinical ethics support (see Fig. 1). The underlying idea is that it makes sense to handle the normative dimensions of clinical encounters (i.e. ethical questions, conflicts, dilemmas) in an "escalation" approach. This strategy suggests that the low-level or "milder" activities are to be exhausted before engaging in higher-level and more directive interventions. In line with our proposal to apply both internal and external standards when evaluating ethics consultation material/activities of colleagues, using this model helps to distinguish between the criteria that are supposed to be shared by the ethics consultant(s) whose work is to be evaluated and those criteria that an observer wants to use as a measure (because such criteria seem to be founded on a large consensus – as in the case of the ASBH core competences).

Finder's narrative in "The Zadeh Scenario" implicitly places his approach – as the authors in Parts Two and Three have vastly agreed – on the so-called "level of conversation with the family and the healthcare professionals," which seems to match the 1st level on Fig. 1; moreover, his approach does not seem to move to any higher level. No explicit clarification of values (2nd level) has been carried out according to the narrative (as several authors have highlighted), nor has any interpretation (3rd level) or analysis (4th level) about the understanding of the value conflict and the options at stake been offered. We assume that these activities (at least levels 1–3, if not 4) would be part of a phenomenological-hermeneutical approach to ethics consultation. For verification of what may serve as Finder's internal standard, we need to look into the way Finder himself explicitly articulated his approach:

> [W]e understand the main activity of ethics consultation as conducting conversations in [...] clinical situations in order to identify by speech, and through oneself as an example, what is most worthwhile to the participants in such conversations. We maintain, moreover, that the aim of clinical ethics consultation is to articulate and examine those possible meanings most prominently evoked within specific situations, which frequently involves identifying the problems perceived by those individuals confronted with a clinical decision, and entails gathering the viewpoints of many different participants included in that decision. All of which means that the method of ethics consultation must be clinical. In summary, clinical ethics consultation has two major characteristics. First, its activities are persistently guided by this question for the consultant, 'What do I need to know?' in order (a) to figure out why a clinical ethics consultation was requested? and (b) to get clear about 'what's going on?' Second, clinical ethics consultants seek to identify and discuss by persistently helping to elicit from *the primary participants* (patient, family, physicians, nurses, and so on) what *they themselves* find troubling and in need of resolution, and therefore what aftermaths they can live with in the light of what is most worthwhile to, and for, them. (Bliton and Finder 1999: 74–5, emphases in the original)

This description clearly shows Finder's conceptual insistence on the activities located on levels 1–3. It also highlights the perspective of the *patient* as a primary concern not only for problem resolution, but in the first place to understand the nature of the problem. If these activities are in accordance with an internal standard, reasons would be needed to explain why parts of this (phenomenological-hermeneutical) clinical ethics repertoire were not used or not shown, e.g. value clarification. It is – we concede – possible that Finder did observe or conclude something that prevented him from following a path that would have appeared more stringent with his internal standard, but we do not see any hints for that in "The Zadeh Scenario," nor in the commentaries.

Using the referred to integrative model (Reiter-Theil 2009), however, does not imply that all levels have to be applied in all situations. The judgment about which steps are to be used has to be made in light of the context of the ethics consultation case. If as in this case the patient's voice appears to have gotten lost, it becomes a normative-ethical claim to make this voice audible, even in a situation of arising resistance (e.g., of the family)(see levels 6, 9 and 10). In some jurisdictions, adopting this claim is a matter of obeying the law and enacting existing ethical guidelines and principles, especially patient rights and respect for autonomy, and as such this normative basis requires the ethics consultant (but also the healthcare professionals)

Table 1 Different evaluation methods and types of material in peer review assessment of EC

Evaluation method	Types of material	Description (types of material)
Analysis of reports (oral or written)	Case vignette	Short, summarizing description of an EC case focusing on the medical situation, the ethical problem and (possible) problem resolution
	Record	Record of an EC, written by a member of the CESS
	Narrative	Detailed narrative of an EC case by a member of the CESS focusing on the author's perspective
	Feedback	Feedback of the patient, relatives or health care providers of an EC
Analysis of videos	Video	Life footage of an (actual or enacted) EC
Embedded research	Observational data, comprehensive report	Case series records, enriched by on-site interviews, structured information, field notes, diary

to work on the identified problem. We hold that this obligation is not even dependent on the (methodological) clinical ethics approach, but is a general duty. However, the style and the steps of how an ethics consultant would try to perform this task will and may vary – according to her approach. Finder, as the author of "The Zadeh Scenario," should (and we believe probably could) explain how he deliberately handled this normative issue. To prevent such gaps of assessment, it is important for the reviewed clinical ethics consultation service and the reviewers to agree in advance about the internal as well as the external standards that are to be utilized in evaluation.

On our review, most of the commentaries in Part Three and their critical reflections on method include the claim that activities corresponding with levels 2–8 in Fig. 1 are missing in "The Zadeh Scenario." We can imagine that several of the authors might even go as far as to request application of steps 9 or 10 in this case, e.g., for enacting the normative claim that the patient's voice and wishes must be made audible (e.g., Armstrong; Aulisio).

To our knowledge, there is no framework referring to different evaluation methods or types of materials used in peer reviewing clinical ethics consultation. A preliminary overview regarding methods and types of materials can be found in Table 1. We share Rasmussen's methodological reservations regarding the suitability of case narratives for peer review. In her thoughtful analysis she makes admirably clear that case narratives do require standardization in order to control for "idiosyncratic framing mechanisms" of their authors – and their readers as well – and for the lack of crucial information. However, using a uniform standardization of case narratives might come with the loss of the specific advantages of narratives, namely to provide a first-person account of the situation. One solution, we suggest, consists in combining a narrative with a more formally structured record in order to compensate the shortcomings of narratives regarding procedural, analytical and normative criteria.

Conclusion

Evaluation of clinical ethics support services – especially clinical ethics consultation – by peer review is an important task on the way towards improving the practice and developing related concepts.

We conclude by listing five core points to consider when evaluating ethics consultation:

- Peer review evaluation of clinical ethics consultation requires application of explicitly articulated external and internal standards both for the doing and for the documentation of ethics consultation. Different criteria may be required for the doing and for the documentation.
- Standardization of criteria is a prerequisite for the evaluation of ethics consultation. Also, the selection and structure of material(s) requested for evaluation should be explicitly standardized. Both requests have to be based on a profession-wide discourse and consensus building as well as on an agreement between those carrying out the evaluation and those whose work is being evaluated.
- In order to balance the weight given to internal and external standards, the use of such standards in the evaluation of ethics consultation should be embedded within a wide, integrative model.
- General obligations – as articulated by law, professional standards, local mores, institutional orientations, communal normative guidelines and principles, and so forth – must be accounted for when establishing an evaluative set of criteria.
- The kinds of material evidence offered for clinical ethics consultation evaluation should be oriented to provide an authentic picture and to avoid gaps of significant information in order to accurately represent the relevant ethical issues of the case.

Acknowledgements We thank Professor Stuart Finder, PhD, for his generous and trusting invitation to contribute to this project of evaluating a case of clinical ethics support. His courage could – maybe should – become a milestone in developing this field further.

References

Agich GJ (2018) Narrative and method in ethics consultation. In: Finder SG, Bliton MJ (eds) Peer review, peer education, and modeling in the practice of clinical ethics consultation: the Zadeh project. Springer, Cham, pp 139–150

American Society for Bioethics and Humanities (2011) Core competencies for healthcare ethics consultation, 2nd edn. American Society for Bioethics and Humanities, Glenview

Armstrong K (2018) Telling about engagement is not enough: seeking the "ethics" of ethics consultation in clinical ethics case reports. In: Finder SG, Bliton MJ (eds) Peer review, peer education and modeling in the practice of clinical ethics consultation. Springer, Cham, pp 63–73

Aulisio MP (2018) (Meta-) methodological lessons for ethics consultation. In: Finder SG, Bliton MJ (eds) Peer review, peer education, and modeling in the practice of clinical ethics consultation: the Zadeh project. Springer, Cham, pp 127–137

Bliton MJ, Finder SG (1999) The peculiar visage of philosophy in clinical ethics consultation. In: Zaner RM (ed) Performance, talk, reflection. What is going on in clinical ethics consultation? Kluwer Academic Publishers, Boston

Bruce CR (2018) Not principlism nor casuistry, not narrative ethics nor clinical pragmatism: a case for proceduralism. In: Finder SG, Bliton MJ (eds) Peer review, peer education, and modeling in the practice of clinical ethics consultation: the Zadeh project. Springer, Cham, pp 113–125

Pfaefflin M, Kobert K, Reiter-Theil S (2009) Evaluating clinical ethics consultation. Camb Q Healthc Ethics 18:406–419

Rasmussen L (2018) Standardizing the case narrative. In: Finder SG, Bliton MJ (eds) Peer review, peer education, and modeling in the practice of clinical ethics consultation: the Zadeh project. Springer, Cham, pp 151–160

Reiter-Theil S (2009) Dealing with the normative dimension in clinical ethics consultation. Camb Q Healthc Ethics 18:347–359

Reiter-Theil S (2012) What does empirical research contribute to medical ethics? a methodological discussion using exemplary studies. Camb Q Healthc Ethics 21:425–435

Reiter-Theil S, Schürmann J (2016) The 'big five' in 100 clinical ethics consultation cases. Evaluating three years of ethics support in the Basel University Hospitals. Bioethica Forum 9(2):12–22

Rubin SB, Zoloft L (eds) (2000) Margin of error. The ethics of mistakes in the practice of medicine. University Publishing, Hagerstown

Schürmann J, Mertz M, Reiter-Theil S (2013) "It is really about arguing?" why clinical ethics support needs metaethics. Unpublished. Poster presentation. International Conference on Clinical Ethics Consultation, March 14–16, 2013, Munich, Germany

Slowther AM, McClimans L, Price C (2012) Development of clinical ethics services in the UK: a national survey. J Med Ethics 38(4):210–214

Doing Well or Doing Good in Ethics Consultation

Jeffrey P. Bishop

Introduction

At one point in history, the medical record was little more than a series of notes written by a doctor to himself. In its original form, it was a short-hand that was mostly idiosyncratic, meant for one set of eyes only. As healthcare became more complex, the chart would need to change. It would become the medium to communicate with other physicians in order to permit coordinated care. It became a document written in a shared language that only a fellow practitioner could understand. Even the patient would never recognize herself in those notes, so distant the medical narrative is from the patient's lived experience.

In time, however, the medical record became the legal record, the official record of what occurred in the interaction of patient with doctor; and perhaps more importantly it became the record of what did not occur. Doctors were suddenly being judged – with severe financial penalties – for what was and was not in their notes. Thus, the medical record changed. It included not only key findings, but it now would also include the absence of key findings that might rule out certain diseases. Doctors had to prove that they had thought of and had ruled out certain diseases. And if we are to believe those lobbying for tort reform, the documentation within the medical record changed the way physicians would practice medicine. Today, the medical record, which is really a legal record, is evolving once again. It has become the record used for billing. Physicians are called by billing abstractors, who ask them questions like: "Did you do this exam or that exam? Because if you did, we could bill at the higher level." "Why, yes," the physician answers, "I did do that exam! So let's bill at the higher rate." This is not to say that the doctors fabricate what goes into

J. P. Bishop (✉)
Albert Gnaegi Center for Health Care Ethics, Saint Louis University, St. Louis, MO, USA
e-mail: jeffrey.bishop@slu.edu

S. G. Finder, M. J. Bliton (eds.), *Peer Review, Peer Education, and Modeling in the Practice of Clinical Ethics Consultation: The Zadeh Project*,
https://doi.org/10.1007/978-3-319-90955-4_13

the chart, because in all likelihood they soon began doing those more highly billable exams. Again, practice can and sometimes does follow documentation.

Having read many medical records, which are also legal and financial records, I was a bit dumbfounded by "The Zadeh Scenario," Finder's narrative of a clinical ethics consultation case that he participated in and submitted for peer-review in these pages. I thought to myself: "Stuart, what are you doing? Don't you know that, given the way you are presenting this case consult, your peer reviewers are going to rake you over the coals?" Of course, Finder knew how the narrative would be engaged by his peers. When Finder approached me to be a part of this project, he told me that he would present a case narrative for peer review, and that he had asked several other colleagues to comment on the peer-reviews. He asked me to provide another layer of commentary onto the commentaries of the peer-reviews. Just to be clear, we need to understand the layers involved here. First, there was the case consultation, the actual doing of the case. Then there is Finder's narrative, "The Zadeh Scenario," a shortened and focused version of what had been done. Then there is the layer of the peer-review commentaries on Finder's narrative of what he had done in the clinical ethics consultation. And then there are the commentaries on the peer-review commentaries of Finder's narrative of the case he had done in the clinical ethics consultation. Within the first lines, I knew that Finder's narrative describing his consult was going to drive his peer-reviewers crazy.

So, why did Finder not give his peer reviewers what they wanted? Finder has been doing clinical ethics since 1991, for well over 25 years at the time this volume was assembled. Having practiced medicine and having practiced clinical ethics consultation, I also know that the chart does not contain everything – every kindness, every word, every smile, every moment of tension – that occurs between a patient and a physician, or a patient and the clinical ethicists. I also feel quite secure in believing that Finder, as a clinical ethics consultant, knows the importance of writing a coherent note in a chart, a note that can be read and understood by clinicians, a note that documents important positive findings, but also negative findings. Certainly, Finder knows that we write with various purposes, highlighting some features of a case over other features of a case. So, why "The Zadeh Scenario"; why this narrative? I think Finder, the clinical ethics consultant, was up to something very interesting when he wrote out this narrative. It was not a narrative fit for review, but a narrative fit for other purposes. The question is whether his peer-reviewers would have ears to hear Finder's rendering of the consult.

From my reading, it turns out his peer-reviewers did not have the ears to hear the story that Finder was telling. They did indeed rake Finder over the coals, as I thought they might. They did so nicely of course; after all, bioethicists are nothing if not nice. Finder knows that his case-narrative is a story about his doing of a consult. He of course knows that his narrative was not the kind of story that his peer-reviewers will have wanted. Rasmussen astutely notes that Finder's rendering of "The Zadeh Scenario" is just that: a rendering of a kind of doing (the doing of clinical ethics consultation) and that all renderings, all telling of stories have a purpose – a point made by Tod Chambers years ago (Rasmussen 2018; Chambers 1999). She notes that absence of evidence in the narrative is not in fact evidence of absence in the consult, despite what lawyers – and it seems clinical ethics peer-reviewers – believe about medical charts.

Finder is pointing to an insight on which Rasmussen picked up: peer-reviewers who would give attestation to quality ethics consultation candidates like Finder will need to be thoughtful about the evidence supplied to them by candidates. More importantly, however, I also think Finder's rendering of the story in just this way calls attention to the special kind of doing that clinical ethics consultation is – a kind of doing that may not fit into what proceduralist ethicists want to see. In this essay – which is now four removes from Finder's actual doing of the case – I shall argue that Finder is not only problematizing the process of attestation of quality, but that he is calling attention to the special kind of doing that is clinical ethics consultation. I shall argue that clinical ethics consultation is a kind of doing that is a local form of moral enquiry, seeking not just to achieve medical – or clinical ethical – goals, but to enact human goods. His peer reviewers want Finder to do clinical ethics well; Finder wants to do good in clinical ethics consultation.

Examining the Commentaries on the Peer-Reviewers' Commentaries of the Narrative of the Doing That Is Clinical Ethics Consultation

Just to be sure we are all on the same page, I am here engaging not the case consult nor the narrative nor the peer reviews of the narrative. I am instead here examining those who commented on the peer-reviews. Bruce claims to see a new methodology emerging in the peer-reviews. Bruce surveys different methods of ethics consultation from principlism to casuistry to narrative to pragmatism. She claims that there might be a new method developing – proceduralism. While she is certainly correct that something new is emerging in clinical ethics consultation, proceduralism is not a new method. Rather, the procedures have been elevated to a normative level by virtue of the fact that clinical ethics consultants desire to have professional standards and it is nice to be able to claim procedural neutrality.

In fact, the proceduralist turn is part of a long history in philosophical ethics in the late modern period. Indeed, the principlist approach is itself a product of that proceduralist turn. Eschewing thick metaphysical moral content – after all no one likes to fight over metaphysics – Beauchamp and Childress claimed that we should turn our attention to the mid-level principles that will assist us in making practical decisions. It matters not, they claimed, whether one held to thick metaphysical moral content of the Catholics or the Methodists, or any other non-religious metaphysical schema: all morally serious people can agree on these mid-level principles (Beauchamp and Childress 2009:. 2–5, 12–14).

However, as H. Tristram Engelhardt noted, Beauchamp and Childress imported too much thick metaphysical moral content under the guise of priniciplism (Engelhardt 1996: 57–58). The principles are merely the philosophical terms given to the kind of procedures that Beauchamp and Childress think will help us to make moral decisions. Engelhardt, in his masterpiece, *The Foundations of Bioethics*, calls for an even thinner proceduralism than that of Beauchamp and Childress, one that focused on forbearance rights and the principle of permission (Engelhardt 1996: 121–123). Likewise, the casuists claimed that Beauchamp and Childress were really still too abstract in their principles, because they are not sufficiently practical, and thus the procedures for doing ethics were still too beholden to abstract philosophy. No one really sits around and tries to trace mid-level abstract principles from the thick metaphysical moral commitments of patients (and of health care systems); they merely repeat what they did in the last case that was similar enough to the case at hand. Thus, casuists claim that the procedures for doing ethics well up from the ground of actual cases and not from mid-level abstract principles, which remain esoteric.

Moreover, when it comes to narrative, Beauchamp and Childress would claim that narrative is completely compatible with their proceduralist ethic (principlism) because patient narratives permit clinical ethicists to specify and balance principles given the patient's values (Beauchamp and Childress 2009: 16–24). Thus, contrary to Bruce's claim that proceduralism is new methodology, it seems clear that proceduralism is at the heart of all four methodologies that she spells out. In fact, the law itself is a proceduralist institution; without appeal to thick metaphysical moral content, it focuses on the proper procedures that should be followed in order to permit people to live their own lives according to their thick moral commitments. Principles, whether derived from thicker metaphysical moral commitments or from similar cases, are part of a proceduralist ethic. Policies are proceduralist. Thus, what Bruce claims to be a new methodology is in fact very old, as old as liberalism itself.

Rasmussen shows us the idiosyncratic requirements of the peer reviewers, telling us that we do not yet have shared procedures for writing up cases for attestation. Each of the peer-reviewers would require different things from Finder's narrative in order for his practice to be declared a good practice. The problem may not be with Finder's practice, but instead the problem might be his narrative choices (Rasmussen 2018: 151). Rasmussen makes her point in the context of discussing Armstrong's feminist critique of Finder's narrative. Finder inexplicably uses the patient's daughters' first names, but he uses "Mr. Zadeh" when referring to the patient's son. However, the discrepancy in reference doesn't give us a full picture of feminist considerations that might have been at play in this consult. There isn't enough evidence to know. The absence of evidence, Rasmussen notes, is not evidence of the absence of feminist concerns in the consult (Rasmussen 2018: 158).

However, Rasmussen's point should be extended to every clinical encounter. The plenum of any encounter, whether clinical or otherwise, can never be captured in any narrative, as Foucault noted (Foucault 1991: ix ff). Every narrative is a selection of what to include, with only the slightest of traces of what gets left out. Every narrative then is already an interpretation of the plenum of experience, and every narrative demands interpretation, because it is already an interpretation.[1]

[1] See Foucault's introduction to *The Birth of the Clinic*, where he notes that there is something about narratives that demand interpretation, that words beget words; interpretations beget interpretation.

Rasmussen's point extends well beyond Finder's use of names in "The Zadeh Scenario." Thus, it is not only true that his peer-reviewers have somewhat idiosyncratic concerns for what Finder ought to report; Finder also chooses what to report and what not to report. Extending Rasmussen's insight, I shall argue that the lack of standards for what should go into narratives for peer-review of clinical ethics consultation is merely a symptom of the problem; it is the surface problem, for we must first figure out exactly what clinical ethics consultation *is* before creating a standard of reporting, lest the *standard of reporting* become the *standard for the practice* of clinical ethics consultation, circumscribing what ought to happen in the practice itself, which precedes the narrative rendering of the plenum of the clinic.

This point is precisely the question taken up by Agich, both in his commentary in these pages and in previous work (see, for example, also Agich 2005, 2009). In his commentary on the peer-reviewers, Agich cites Alasdair MacIntyre's definition of a practice:

> A practice may be identified as a set of considerations, manners, uses, observances, customs, standards, canons, maxims, principles, rules and offices specifying useful procedures or denoting obligations or duties which relate to human actions and utterances. It is ... an adverbial qualification of choices and performances, more or less complicated in which conduct is understood in terms of a procedure. Words such as punctually, considerately, civilly, scientifically, legally, candidly, judicially, poetically, morally, etc., do not specify performances; they postulate performances and specify *procedural conditions* to be taken into account when choosing and acting. (Agich 2018: 139; emphasis added by Agich)

Agich gets it right on rules/procedures vs. the enactment of – indeed embodiment of – rules and procedures. Agich continues: "The rules involved in ethics consultation are first and foremost enacted and are phenomenologically manifested in and through the actions, cognitions, and perceptions of consultants" (Agich 2018: 142). Yet, Agich warns clinical ethicists to be careful about deploying rules.

> The rules are not and cannot be reduced to a formal code or set of guidelines or procedures that might be followed like a recipe. Instead, the rules, even when articulated linguistically, as they certainly must be for various legitimate purposes, are just abstractions from the lived experience of the practice and, importantly, they are dependent upon that practice for their ultimate meaning and justification. In this sense, statements about ethics consultation methodology and theories of ethics consultation are *secondary* to the actual practice itself. (Agich 2018: 142)

The peer-reviewers would reduce the practice to the practice of following the guidelines. Virtually all the authors in Parts Two and Three, with the exception of Rosell & Johnson, and to a lesser extent Hynds, are applying abstract rules to the case. First, figure out what clinical ethics consultants do (Chidwick et al. 2010; Frolic and Rubin 2018) and then generalize it to be applicable beyond the case at hand (Frolic and Rubin 2018; Tarzian 2018; Bruce 2018). These are the abstractions – now not from theories, but abstracts from particular cases – that become the codes, procedures, and policies to now be applied by ethicists to all cases. Agich is warning clinical ethics consultants to be very careful.

Yet, even Agich misses something important that MacIntyre also says about practices. MacIntyre notes that practices are not just a simple form of doing; they are in fact very complex, because all true practices are aimed at something that not one peer-reviewer or one commentator mentioned: practices are aimed at goods. MacIntyre states:

> By a practice, I am going to mean any coherent and complex form of socially established cooperative human activity through which goods internal to that form of activity are realised in the course of trying to achieve those standards of excellence which are appropriate to, and partially definitive of that form of activity, with the result that human powers to achieve excellence, and human conceptions *to the ends and goods involved*, are systematically extended. (MacIntyre 1984 p. 187 [emphasis added])

Thus, planting seeds is not a practice, but farming is. Throwing a ball is not a practice, but baseball is.

I would argue that if clinical ethics consultation is a practice, it has to have normative goods toward which it aims. What are the goods of clinical ethics consultation? I do not mean the *goals*, but rather the *goods*. Are those goods allied with medical goods? How are they different from medical goods? From whence do the goods come?

First, as Agich discusses, we must focus on the actual doing of clinical ethics, not on the procedures which are post-hoc derivations from practice, or prescriptions by so-called experts. Tyrannies of proceduralism can arise from the bottom up or from the top down. When doing clinical ethics, a master practitioner is not just following a set of rules. She enacts, enlivens, indeed embodies the rules such that they are not mere rules applied, but have become actions aimed at goods. It is even odd to refer to them as embodied rules or procedures at all. She knows which rules to follow and which to reject. She knows which guidelines and policies are unnecessary and which guidelines or policies are indeed made ridiculous given the particulars of an encounter. That means that, second, the rules cannot and should not be reduced to a formal code. The rules, guidelines, processes, policies, and procedures are not formulae to be followed. The rules, guidelines, processes, policies, and procedures are codified for other purposes, which are tangentially important to the actual doing of clinical ethics. I shall return to this point a little later, but before I do I want to turn our attention to the peer-reviewers themselves.

A Commentary on the Peer-Review Commentaries of the Narrative of the Doing That Is Clinical Ethics Consultation

Finder begins "The Zadeh Scenario" (which is an interpretative summary of the actual consult) *in media res*, the action already afoot. In fact, the narrative begins with the concluding statement of a family whose mother has been in the hospital for weeks and sick for several years. Of course, peer-reviewers would prefer to have things begin at the beginning and to end at the ending. By beginning in the middle, Finder already disrupts the procedural flow that his peer-reviewers expect. Who initiated the consult, and for what purposes was it initiated? Several commentators (Hynds 2018) noted that beginnings always matter in case consults. But do they really? That may be where one wants a narrative to begin, but consults themselves are mired in the middle of the ongoing action, in the midst of the plenum. Everyone in medicine also knows that all consultants – clinical ethics consultants or medical consultants – like to have a delimited question. What does the requestor of the consult want the consultant to address? Thus, as Hynds points out, getting the question right is of first importance, and most assuredly Hynds is correct. Of course, Finder knows that getting the question delimited is of first importance; but he does not begin "The Zadeh Scenario" in this way. He does not lay out the value conflict for his peer-reviewers to see it very clearly, because in the actual doing of a consult it is often the case that the value conflict has not yet emerged, even while the clinicians caught up in the midst of the plenum may feel the resultant uneasiness. Much of the time, the request for a consult emerges because something does not feel right. In this case, it was the family that did not feel things were right. Finder is pointing to the fact that the clinical ethics consultant is the mid-wife bringing forth into clarity the uneasiness felt by those in the midst of the action.[2]

Every clinical ethics consultant – including Finder – knows that the first order of business is to establish the stakeholders, gathering their views on the case. Of course, the most important stakeholder is the patient. Many of the reviewers note that Ms. Hamadani is missing from "The Zadeh Scenario" (Frolic and Rubin 2018; Armstrong 2018; Tarzian 2018; Rosell and Johnson 2018). How could Finder have missed this? Of course, absence of evidence in the narrative is not in fact evidence of absence in the consult, as I (and Rasmussen) have already noted. Still, as tort law has taught medicine, naming absences is of utmost importance when regulating behaviors.

Yet, perhaps attuning to what matters, attuning to the particulars, Finder already knew that Ms. Hamadani could not participate in the conversation about her care. Finder, attuning to what matters – as all good consultants do – turns to the family, who are present and are actively engaged and are concerned. But to the hermeneutics of suspicion that tends to accompany the individualism regnant in American culture, something is strange about the zealotry of the family's concern (as Armstrong points out). Why didn't Finder's narrative tell his peer-reviewers that the family did indeed have the patient's best interests at heart? After all, one of them was at Ms. Hamadani's bedside night and day. Or could it be that ethics consultants are really just Western individualists who are always suspicious of family-members meddling in the individual patient's business? Surely, Finder knows that he should have bowed his head to autonomy, and traced out whether the patient had advance directives, powers of attorney, stated preferences – all the legal procedures meant to create the kinds of freedoms important in clinical ethics consultation.

[2] By bringing forth, I am meaning something akin to what Heidegger means in *The Question Concerning Technology* (1993 pp. 307–342). Technology challenges forth what it desires from the world, where Heidegger notes that in a *techne* something is brought forth.

Of course, clinical ethics consultants are always looking out for the best interests of patients. Finder points out that the patient is Persian. In fact, she is from Iran and is a traditionalist like her youngest daughter (Finder 2018: 33). Tarzian praises Finder for bringing up this important fact. She even notes the importance of the Persian concept of *T'aarof,* "a ritual politeness code that governs behaviors between individuals of different hierarchies and imposes obligations to mitigate emotional distress by way of avoiding negative feelings through specific culturally-engrained social etiquette" (Tarzian 2018: 78). Clinical ethics consultants should always demonstrate their cultural competency, an important indicator that they are not deploying colonial power structures on their patients, permitting patients to have their own ethical value systems; unless, of course, those ethical value systems and hierarchies violate Western understandings of individualism and autonomy. After all, ethics consultants are there mostly to deal in value conflicts, and clearly knowing the patient's values from the patient's own mouth would go a long way to be sure there were no conflicts between family members and to alleviate the distress of those who do clinical ethics consultation.

Yet, it seems to me that Finder mediated the case very nicely, mostly by listening and reflecting what was said back to the family. Finder did not intervene to *do* anything, prompting several of the peer reviewers to ask whether this was an ethics consultation at all. (Hynds 2018) I would argue Finder's peer-reviewers questioned this precisely *because* Finder's narrative had not documented the procedures. In short, Finder's narrative gave no attention to the typical things that his expert peer-reviewers would want to see. That is because Finder's narrative focused more on the kind of doing that clinical ethics consultation is as opposed to focusing on the procedures that the experts would want to see.

Thus, while I agree with Rasmussen that we must understand exactly what goes into an appropriate narrative for peer review, I also think that we should reflect upon the kind of doing that clinical ethics consultation is, a doing that exceeds any narrative documentation, including procedural narrative documentation. Put differently, the peer-reviewers have already committed the error against which Agich warns us, namely that deploying the procedures and following them with rote vigor renders the doing of ethics more like planting seeds than like the practice of farming. In short, they are focused on doing clinical ethics consultation well. As such, his peer-reviewers kept judging him as if he were merely planting seeds. But Finder was doing something more akin to farming; accordingly, Finder was focused on doing good in clinical ethics consultation.

A Commentary on the Narrative of the Doing That Is Clinical Ethics Consultation

It is important to understand that Finder belongs to the philosophical tradition of phenomenology. Phenomenology is itself a kind of methodology within philosophy. It begins with Edmund Husserl, who himself was attempting to ground science

(Husserl 1970).[3] On one hand, science had been caught between two philosophical ways of grounding understanding – rationalism and empiricism; this scientific grounding, because it had eschewed metaphysics, collapsed science into a positivism – where scientists began to think that they could have a one-to-one correspondence between a word and a thing. On the other hand, because science could not ground its knowledge in the world, Nietzschean irrationalism took hold, where reason had become a mask for power relations. Husserl held that if we could bracket our plain everyday stances toward the world – which are often mistaken – and attune to the things as they appear to us, we might ground science. Out of that bracketing, Husserl argues, we might be able to give an account of the eidetic features of experience so that we can ground science in intersubjective experience, which is a kind of very careful peer review. Thus, science need not be secured in rationalism or empiricism, nor in positivism. Nor does it succumb, Husserl thinks, to irrationalism.

Husserl's insights went way beyond securing science; in fact, his phenomenological methodology gave birth to several philosophical insights about the nature of existential experience, ethical experience, embodied experience, among many other aspects of human experience.[4] Richard Zaner – a major figure in the American phenomenological tradition – can be credited for bringing phenomenology into the clinical ethics arena. Finder's practice of clinical ethics consultation is greatly informed by Zaner.[5]

One of the things that phenomenology asks us to do is to bracket our preconceptions – even our procedural preconceptions – about what we think matters in a case, and to attend to the things that matter to the patient, to the patient's family, and to the patient's caregivers. It asks us to pay attention to contexts and spaces and times and situations, and how those contribute to our perceptions of what matters. Because patient concerns are idiosyncratic and highly particular, we must bracket universalizing theories, whether those be deontological or utilitarian, or our cultural notions of liberalism or proceduralism. We must bracket our theories of autonomy and understand the way actual, particular people conceive themselves, which usually happens to be in contextual relationships of families, contrary to the dogmas of individualism, upon which Western bioethics – including clinical ethics – is built.

What Finder does with "The Zadeh Scenario" defies the typical framing of clinical ethics consultants, who are bent on procedures and Western ideals of individualism. Finder offers us what he has judged mattered in the case, not what most clinical ethicists think should have mattered to him. What ethics consultants think matters floats above all cases and seems to emerge from no particular case. Is it not possible

[3] Actually, many philosophers think that phenomenology begins with Aristotle, but that point is unimportant for what follows.

[4] Husserl started many philosophers off on many different trajectories, for example, Martin Heidegger, Emmanuel Levinas, Alfred Schutz, Edith Stein, Hannah Arendt, Jean-Paul Sartre, and Maurice Merleau-Ponty just to name a few.

[5] Finder, hired by Zaner and then serving as his colleague for the final 11 years of Zaner's career at Vanderbilt University Medical Center, was also mentored by Zaner – and the two remain personal friends.

that in the careful attunement of Finder's phenomenological reduction, he figured out that the patient was too gravely ill to participate in decision-making? Or perhaps through the reduction, he recognized immediately that the patient wanted her family to take all decisions on her behalf, because that is how a Persian family shows love in their particular cultural context. Shouldn't "The Zadeh Scenario" have just said so, then? No, not if Finder wanted to highlight other features that are more important to the actual doing of this particular case.

Or perhaps "The Zadeh Scenario" is an act of opposition, a subtle commentary on Western bioethicists. After all, Finder kindly, gently, and subtly chastises Dr. Moore's somewhat more aggressive adherence to hospital procedures. Moore constantly presents the question of code status repeatedly to the family, driving them to question his motives, asking that Moore no longer be the ethics consultant on Ms. Hamadani's case at all. It seems to me that Finder is saying that any of the peer-reviewers would have been drummed out of the room as well given their procedural concerns.

Finder's telling in "The Zadeh Scenario" is pointing to what was going on with a particular family, who lived and moved and had their being within a particular culture with its own particular rich resources for problem solving. Finder is pointing to the fact that this family was asking everyone not to prejudge. This family was asking everyone to bracket their concerns and to attune to this particular family's concerns. Finder points out that the family did not want anyone to prejudge the situation with their mother: they did not want the consulting doctors to prejudge; they did not want Dr. Moore to prejudge; and as Finder's narrative points out, they did not even want Finder – or any other clinical ethics consultant – to prejudge. This family indicates repeatedly that they know what is really happening with their mother in the excess of their experience with their mother. The weight of their mother's dying did not need the added pressure of proceduralists wanting clear directives. They knew all along that they would not ask for CPR when the time came. However, for whatever reason, that could not be said by them or to them until that time arrived.

Finder's participation was not, therefore, necessarily without warrant; this family might have needed him for another purpose: to act as witness and perhaps even midwife, bringing forth what really mattered to them. And this is what "The Zadeh Scenario" repeatedly shows us, i.e., what matters to the family, and that the doing of clinical ethics consultation might mean that the ethics consultant's prejudgments need to be bracketed so that she can attend to what matters to the patient in the moment, and if not the patient, then those who love the patient and have repeatedly demonstrated it.

In fact, "The Zadeh Scenario" is a narrative of what matters to the patient and the family. This narrative is a narrative describing the bringing forth of goods possible in dying. With this narrative, Finder challenges us to bracket our procedures and policies and guidelines. Finder even describes his own marginalization. Dr. Brouhkims turns to Finder essentially asking him to endorse what he and the family have enacted. Finder does so, rather uncomfortably, and the family has to assert once again, that they know what is happening, and what decisions must be taken to do right by their mother. They do not even need Finder.

So, "The Zadeh Scenario" has a purpose. The purpose seems to be two-fold. First, it is a phenomenological account of what matters to a particular family caring for a particular patient with all of the attendant idiosyncrasies. What matters is highly dependent upon the particularities of a case, particularities that do not admit of the generalizations – of the abstractions – of the policies and procedures of clinical ethics consultation. The second purpose of is to highlight the kind of doing that clinical ethics consultation is. It draws our attention to the doing of clinical ethics consultation by marginalizing the clinical ethics consultant. Finder notes that he is bearing witness; but bearing witness to what? I believe it is to the kind of doing that clinical ethics consultants have not really begun to understand, especially those who would judge the practice according to a set of pre-conceived standards, by which all ethics consultants are to be judged – the attestation procedures.

Conclusion (The Kind of Doing That Is Clinical Ethics Consultation)

I have pointed out above that clinical ethics consultation is a practice and that practices are aimed at goods, and not merely at goals. All but one peer-reviewer of "The Zadeh Scenario" mentioned goals, sometimes in terms of goals of care, sometimes as the goals of ethics or ethical goals. Not a single essay, whether those of the second-level commentators or the first-level peer-reviewers, used the terms "goods," "goods of care," or even "the goods of medicine." Clinicians know that goals are important for the practice that is medicine. But everyone seems to avoid the question of the goods of medicine, let alone speaking of the goods of clinical ethics consultation. We have to go back to the writings of Edmund Pellegrino to find a sustained treatment on the goods of medicine (Pellegrino 2008:147–159). People do not seek out medicine because it has goals, but because it has goods that they desire for their lives, goods that they want embodied. In fact, those of us who sought to become nurses or physicians – and even those of us who desired to become clinical ethics consultants – did so because we thought that through these practices we were pursuing goods for patients, not merely goals. Planting is a goal-directed activity; farming is aimed at bringing forth goods – fruits and vegetables. Planting seeds is a procedure; growing fruits is a practice. Procedures that might help us do well at clinical ethics consultation might get in the way of doing good through clinical ethics consultation. So, here we have it: in order to be a practice, clinical ethics consultants must pursue goods, not goals.

Buried inside "The Zadeh Scenario" are the goods of clinical ethics. Those goods are subjective, idiosyncratically named and defined by patients, embedded in an institution of health care that purports to be of service to the goods of health. The clinical ethics consultant, at her best, acts as a careful mid-wife, attempting to bring forth the goods desired, the goods possible, and perhaps even the goods that are not possible for patients. After all, some goods pursued by patients are not possible due to the limits of medicine. Some goods pursued by medicine are not desired by patients. Some goods pursued by clinical ethicists might be limited and provisional, like the desire to limit clinical ethicists to doing what the guidelines and procedures say. Some things thought to be goods by anyone involved in healthcare may not be good at all. "The Zadeh Scenario" acts to problematize the goals of clinical ethics consultation, asking it to focus on the goods that the practice might bring forth.

I occasionally travel to Rome. When in Rome, I often stay with the Irish Dominicans of San Clemente near the Colosseum, on via Lubicana. And since I love to walk, I often walk everywhere I go. If you walk west along via Lubicana passing to the north of the Colosseum you end up on the Via dei Fori Imperiali, which runs up to the Piazza Venezia which is essentially a huge intersection and roundabout in front of the monument to Vittorio Emanuele.[6]

Hundreds of pedestrians attempt to cross the intersection/roundabout while an endless stream of cars and buses enter and exit. There is even a large bus stop at one of the roundabout entrances. So hundreds of cars, buses and pedestrians are all crossing at once. There are no lights, no walk signs. Everyone is crossing and driving and hesitating and starting and stopping. To my American mind and to my North Atlantic desire for rules and laws to govern even the simplest of intersections, that roundabout seems utterly chaotic and dangerous.

To the Romans and those immersed in a kind of personalist culture, the chaos is ordered by the subtlest reading of faces and movement. The drivers are watching facial and bodily expressions of the pedestrians. The Roman pedestrians are watching the drivers of busses and cars. There are no rules and procedures; or rather the rules and procedures are embodied, and thus can only be called rules or procedures in a highly abstract, post-hoc way.

Foreign pedestrians in time come to see what the locals are doing. The Roman pedestrians look to see what the drivers are doing. They see that the drivers are looking to see what the pedestrians are doing. The Roman pedestrians read the movement of the cars and the faces of the drivers. The drivers are reading the bodily expressions and faces of the pedestrians. There is an informal turn-taking between pedestrians and drivers. In short, these pedestrians and drivers see what an American cannot see in the subtlest of movement – a tilted head, a nod, a nonchalant wave of a finger, a gesture. And it all works. It is a different way of interacting from the Anglo-Germanic way and from the American proceduralist way of interacting.

With "The Zadeh Scenario," Finder is depicting a phenomenological – indeed a personalist – engagement; he is trying to read the subtle clues given by the physicians and nurses, and the patient and the patient's family, subtleties that slip through the coarse sieve that is proceduralism. He is trying to get across the roundabout/intersection, or perhaps better, he is trying to help a family of pedestrians navigate

[6] I am not dropping names here or attempting show off how cultured I am. The details matter and I suspect that these details seem foreign to the reader, which is precisely the point. But they are details that challenge our settled visions about intersections.

the complexity, walking them across the roundabout/intersection. But he has to know where they want to go, and whether crossing here is the right place to cross to get there. He is helping them to read the subtle clues of the drivers and other pedestrians, paying attention to what matters – to what is the matter at hand – rather than to the rules articulated by proceduralists. But Finder has to know what the goods are that his practice is trying to enable. He has to know how the goods of clinical ethics consultation are related to the goods of medicine, and how the goods of medicine might enable (or disable) the goods of a patients. He has to focus on the doing of clinical ethics, which is a kind of bringing forth of goods. That is the primary kind of doing that is clinical ethics consultation.

Clinical ethics consultation is, as I have argued (with colleagues) elsewhere, a kind of particularist and local form of moral enquiry; it is a kind of non-rule governed floundering about (Bishop et al. 2009). The peer-reviewers of "The Zadeh Scenario" are kind of like me – standing at the roundabout in Rome waiting for a light to turn, or for traffic to stop, claiming that these Romans don't know what they are doing. "Finder should wait to cross until there is a light… oh, there are no lights. Well then we should put some lights in here, because how can anyone know what to do." Meanwhile, a family has been asked to make their decisions about when to cross the roundabout/intersection on their own, and Finder now realizes that he must bear witness to the fact that they did not need his help after all; they just needed some time away from the people telling them how to cross the intersection. Finder's peer reviewers want to do well at the process of clinical ethics consultation; Finder in "The Zadeh Scenario" is trying to do good in clinical ethics consultation. The difference is an important one on which clinical ethicists should reflect.

References

Agich GJ (2005) What kind of doing is ethics consultation? Theor Med Bioeth 26(1):7–24

Agich GJ (2009) Clinical ethics as practice. J Int Bioethique 20(4):15–24

Agich GJ (2018) Narrative and method in ethics consultation. In: Finder SG, Bilton MJ (eds) Peer review, peer education, and modeling in the practice of clinical ethics consultation: the Zadeh project. Springer, Cham, pp 139–150

Armstrong K (2018) Telling about engagement is not enough: seeking the "ethics" of ethics consultation in clinical ethics case reports. In: Finder SG, Bilton MJ (eds) Peer review, peer education, and modeling in the practice of clinical ethics consultation: the Zadeh project. Springer, Cham, pp 63–73

Beauchamp TL, Childress JF (2009) Principles in biomedical ethics, 6th edn. Oxford University Press, New York

Bishop JP, Fanning JB, Bliton MJ (2009) Of goals and goods and floundering about: a Dissensus report on clinical ethics consultation. HEC Forum 21(3):275–291

Bruce CR (2018) Not principlism nor casuistry, not narrative ethics nor clinical pragmatism: a case for proceduralism. In: Finder SG, Bilton MJ (eds) Peer review, peer education, and modeling in the practice of clinical ethics consultation: the Zadeh project. Springer, Cham, pp 113–125

Chambers T (1999) The fiction of bioethics. Routledge, New York

Chidwick P, Bell J, Connolly E, Coughlin MD, Frolic AN, Hardingham L, Zlotnik Shaul R (2010) Exploring a model role description for ethicists. HEC Forum 22:31–40

Engelhardt HT Jr (1996) The foundations of bioethics, 2nd edn. Oxford University Press, New York
Finder SG (2018) The Zadeh scenario. In: Finder SG, Bilton MJ (eds) Peer review, peer education, and modeling in the practice of clinical ethics consultation: the Zadeh project. Springer, Cham, pp 21–42
Foucault M (1991) The birth of the clinic: archaeology of medical perception. Translated by A. M. Sheridan Smith. Vintage Books, New York. Originally published in 1963 as Naissance de la clinique by Presses Universitaires de France
Frolic A, Rubin S (2018) Critical self-reflection as moral practice: a collaborative meditation on peer review in ethics consultation. In: Finder SG, Bilton MJ (eds) Peer review, peer education, and modeling in the practice of clinical ethics consultation: the Zadeh project. Springer, Cham, pp 47–61
Heidegger M (1993) The question concerning technology. In: Krell DF (ed) Basic writings. Harper Collins, New York
Husserl E (1970) The crisis of European sciences and transcendental phenomenology. Translated by David Carr. Northwestern University Press, Evanston
Hynds J (2018) Ethics consultation, professional praxis, and what it means to be a "consultant". In: Finder SG, Bilton MJ (eds) Peer review, peer education, and modeling in the practice of clinical ethics consultation: the Zadeh project. Springer, Cham, pp 85–97
MacIntyre A (1984) After virtue, 2nd edn. University of Notre Dame Press, Notre Dame
Pellegrino PD. 2008. The philosophy of medicine reborn: a Pellegrino reader. H. Tristram Engelhardt, Jr Fabrice Jotterand. Notre Dame: University of Notre Dame Press
Rasmussen L (2018) Standardizing the case narrative. In: Finder SG, Bilton MJ (eds) Peer review, peer education, and modeling in the practice of clinical ethics consultation: the Zadeh project. Springer, Cham, pp 151–160
Rosell T, Johnson B (2018) This may, or may not, be an ethics consultation. In: Finder SG, Bilton MJ (eds) Peer review, peer education, and modeling in the practice of clinical ethics consultation: the Zadeh project. Springer, Cham, pp 99–107
Tarzian A (2018) Ethics consultation for Ms. Hamadani: a focus on process. In: Finder SG, Bilton MJ (eds) Peer review, peer education, and modeling in the practice of clinical ethics consultation: the Zadeh project. Springer, Cham, pp 75–84

Peer Review and Beyond: Towards a Dialogical Approach of Quality in Ethics Support

Guy A. M. Widdershoven, Bert Molewijk, and Suzanne Metselaar

Introduction

This unique book provides an open, sensitive and enriching insight into what peer review of clinical ethics support can look like and how peer review can reflect on the quality of a concrete clinical ethics consultation. It is based on a thick description of an ethics consultation, written by an ethics consultant. The book consists of several layers: within each layer, peer-review is organized in a different way and with a different focus. First, five colleagues review the case consultation itself, addressing its strong and weak points. Next, four ethicists reflect on the methods used within both the case consultation and the five initial reviews of the case. In this chapter, we comment on the conclusions of the five initial reviews and the four reflections of the methods used, adding another layer to the reflection process.

We will first go into the relevance of peer review for assessing the quality of clinical ethics consultation. We will argue that peer review in the narrative form as

G. A. M. Widdershoven (✉)
Department of Medical Humanities, VU University Medical Center,
Amsterdam, The Netherlands
e-mail: g.widdershoven@vumc.nl

B. Molewijk
Department of Medical Humanities, VU University Medical Center,
Amsterdam, The Netherlands

Centre of Medical Ethics, University of Oslo, Oslo, Norway
e-mail: a.molewijk@vumc.nl

S. Metselaar
Amsterdam Public Health research institute, VU University Medical Center,
Amsterdam, The Netherlands
e-mail: s.metselaar1@vumc.nl

S. G. Finder, M. J. Bliton (eds.), *Peer Review, Peer Education, and Modeling in the Practice of Clinical Ethics Consultation: The Zadeh Project*,
https://doi.org/10.1007/978-3-319-90955-4_14

presented in this book provides an alternative to the formal clinical ethics consultation review procedures typically found in the clinical ethics literature. Subsequently, drawing on the four chapters on method, we will elaborate on peer review as a reflection on clinical ethics consultation practice (addressed by Agich and Bruce), the elements which a story should contain in order to provide a basis for peer review (discussed by Agich and Aulisio), and the differences between the assessments of the peer reviewers (highlighted by Bruce and Rasmussen). Next, we will argue that a narrative approach to assessing the quality of ethics consultation can be further developed by allowing all stakeholders who are involved in the clinical ethics practice to actively take part in the evaluation process, following a "responsive evaluation" approach. An example of this is creating a Community of Practice, the aim of which is to foster a joint learning process of all parties involved. At the end of this chapter, we draw some conclusions on peer review as a dialogical tool for evaluating quality of clinical ethics consultation.

The Relevance of Peer Review for Assessing the Quality of CES

Clinical ethics support services (CESS) has become broadly accepted in many countries over the past 30 years. Bringing together ethicists and health care professionals trained in ethics, its aim is to contribute to the quality of healthcare. Typically, this is accomplished by having clinical ethics consultants interact with physicians and other healthcare professionals, patients and families, and others directly involved in the care of patients in order to provide input – by fostering deliberation, by asking questions, or by giving case or policy recommendations – into what are often crucial decisions and processes. Although the comprehensive and sustained study of the effects of CES – and especially clinical ethics consultation – is still in its infancy, there is evidence from practice and research that clinical ethics consultation is often experienced as meaningful and relevant by the parties involved (Slowther et al. 2001; Fox et al. 2007; Førde et al. 2008; Molewijk et al. 2008a, b; Pedersen et al. 2009; Førde and Pedersen 2011; Lillemoen and Pedersen 2013; Janssens et al. 2015; Weidema et al. 2015; Svantesson et al. 2014). However, this evidence for the meaningfulness and relevance of clinical ethics consultation does not guarantee that the ethics consultation itself was of a good quality. Therefore, the question of how best to assess the quality of clinical ethics consultation deserves further attention. At issue are such matters as: How to determine, both empirically and theoretically, the quality of ethics consultation? What are characteristics of good ethics consultation? Which elements are necessary? How should the quality of ethics consultation be evaluated? Who should evaluate the quality of ethics consultation? Which methods or measures should be used? Such questions are important, especially because clinical ethics consultation presents itself as a reflective practice in relation to ethical issues in healthcare institutions. At the heart of ethics consultation is the focus on how to determine and define 'quality'. Therefore, we agree with Agich that clinical ethics consultation should also reflect upon its own activities.

In response to questions concerning the quality of ethics consultation, professionals in the field have taken initiatives, for instance by describing the core competencies of ethics consultants (e.g., ASBH 2011), by developing educational programs (La Puma and Schiedermayer 1991; Spike 2012; Dorries et al. 2014; Stolper et al. 2015), and by developing guidelines and protocols (Reiter-Theil 2009; Pedersen et al. 2010; Tarzian et al. 2015; Molewijk et al. 2015; Pearlman et al. 2016). Emphasis has been placed on both procedural aspects (what steps to follow during the consultation, how to make a report, how to evaluate the consultation and take care of follow up, etc.), and on content (how to delineate the ethical issue at stake, which method of analysis is to be used, which aspects should be taken into account in the deliberation, etc.).

Despite their value, most of these initiatives remain abstract and procedural in describing (conditions for) quality of ethics consultation: they focus on the quality of CESS staff, CESS structures/groups and clinical ethics procedures. They often entail formal prescriptions of what *should* be done instead of a thick and narrative description on what *is actually* done in clinical ethics practice. Moreover, core competencies, guidelines and protocols for quality of ethics consultation tend to be used in a deductive way, applying a certain framework of definitions, criteria and norms. This does not allow for a more interactive, critical and reflective process for examining quality of ethics consultation in the context of actual clinical ethics consultation practice. Peer review, on the other hand, is such a process.

For our purposes here, by "peer review "we mean the evaluation of one's work by qualified members of a profession within the relevant field (peers). Peer review is thus a form of self-regulation used to maintain quality standards, improve performance, and provide credibility. For a large part, the work presented in this book is concerned with this kind of self-regulatory quality assessment; utilizing "The Zadeh Scenario," Finder's narrative of the Zadeh case, the central question that is being explored is this: how and on which grounds do peers evaluate the quality of the work of a clinical ethicist?

In particular, Finder's initiative and effort to describe a case consultation in detail and to ask for different kinds of review from peers of different clinical ethics backgrounds stimulates a series of in-depth reflections at several levels. One general conclusion that appears to be shared by all commentators is that peer review should go beyond checking whether clinical ethics staff is adequately educated, guidelines are known or protocols are present. Of crucial importance are the attention for details and the sensitivity for how facts in the case (e.g. behavior, words used, medical situation) are interpreted and valued by both the stakeholders within the specific clinical ethics consultation and for the individual clinical ethics consultant. This hermeneutic sensitivity relates both to the consultation process itself and to the way in which it is reviewed by peers. Another conclusion which is generally shared by the commentators is that peer review requires openness, vulnerability and willingness to learn. This goes beyond a formal attitude of accounting for ethics consultation procedures.

Peer Review as a Reflection on CES Practice

According to Agich, clinical ethics consultation is a practice with implicit standards and rules. Following Schön, Agich argues that clinical ethics professionals are and should be reflective practitioners, and that reflection is needed in order to prevent routinization. Peer review can foster this process of reflection by focusing on the rules which are inherent in the practice of clinical ethics consultation. This is not a theoretical matter of first identifying basic principles of quality of ethics consultation and then investigating whether a certain clinical ethics practice adheres to them, but a practical matter of discovering, or exploring the ways in which what might be called "implicit" standards and rules are enacted in clinical ethics practice. A narrative which presents the concrete experiences of an ethics consultant can therefore provide material for peer review and help the peer reviewer to understand the issues at stake in clinical ethics practice. This we see in the appreciation of "The Zadeh Scenario" by the other authors in this book. They are interested in what the narrative tells about the clinical ethicist's practice and are keen to learn from the experiences which Finder shares with the reader. Despite the fact that a narrative is never complete, the narrative form itself evokes reflection and enables us to understand and reflect upon quality of ethics consultation.

Like Agich, Bruce also recognizes the interest of the peer reviewers in the intricacies of Finder's story. She notices that the reviewers hardly refer to accepted methods of ethical analysis, like principlism and casuistry, to assess the quality of the ethical consultation presented in the story. Accordingly, Bruce regards both the story and the reviews as examples of a narrative and clinical pragmatist approach to clinical ethics consultation, and she applauds the fact that the peer reviews of the Zadeh case are practical and process-oriented rather than theory-driven: "*their methods are interpersonal in nature, one involving an interpretative process or a deliberate uncovering of ethical meanings. A common feature that undergirds all of their assessments seems to be an implicit belief that engaging in patient care entails finding a clinically-feasible (but process-driven) solution*" (Bruce 2018: 114). Hence, Bruce appreciates the pragmatist and intersubjective nature of this kind of peer review.

Both Agich and Bruce, therefore, are drawing explicit attention to the fact that the quality of ethics consultation as a practice can only be assessed by reflecting on the experiences and actions of the ethical consultant, and that a narrative form is of crucial importance.

A Focus on Dealing with Ethical Issues

Although both the peer reviewers in Part Two and the commentators in Part Three are positive about the use of narratives to provide insight into the practice of clinical ethics consultation, they also are critical of "The Zadeh Scenario" in particular, mainly because it does not tell much about Finder's actions as an *ethicist*.

According to Agich, the story Finder presents does not provide information about the way in which the consultant addressed and analyzed relevant values and norms of participants. The story does show the process of consultation, especially the communication in the consultation team, the importance of consultation service records, and the dynamic character of the consultation. As such it provides useful information for peer review. Yet, it lacks reflection on the role of the consultant as ethicist and the analytical and reflective actions of the ethicist. According to Agich, the story is inadequate in this respect, and the commentaries of the peer reviewers make this clear.

Like Agich, Aulisio too highlights information that is missing in "The Zadeh Scenario" as pertinent to core elements of ethics consultation. From the missing information, he draws three lessons, stating what core elements of ethics consultation should entail. First, ethics consultation needs to identify and analyze value conflicts. Second, it should focus on fostering an adequate distribution of responsibilities, and establish who has authority over decision-making. And third, it should, while recognizing the needs of family, keep a focus on the patient. In drawing out these core elements of clinical ethics practice, Aulisio critically evaluates both the narrative Finder presents and the clinical ethics practice presented by that narrative. According to him, both reflect a lacking or absence of key elements necessary for what he considers to be "good" clinical ethics consultation practice.

What we can learn from Agich and Aulisio is that a narrative may only serve as a vehicle for peer review if what it shows is *how* the ethics consultant addressed *ethical* issues. The narrative, thus, should focus on the identification of ethical elements of a clinical situation, the analysis of values and norms of the stakeholders involved in that clinical situation, and the way in which value conflicts are made explicit and turned into an issue for deliberation.

Differences Between Assessments

A pertinent feature of this book is not only that it presents a series of peer reviews but that there is real difference between the assessments of the peer reviewers. In referring to these differences, Bruce highlights the relevance of a procedural approach when assessing not merely Finder's consultation but the quality of ethics consultation more generally. This is in line with the traditional focus on competencies, protocols and guidelines when assessing and warranting quality of clinical ethics services; similar focus can be found in current approaches to quality management in healthcare as a whole. Rasmussen too clearly argues for standards. She sees in the lack of congruence between the peer reviewers a need for a more standardized approach, both for clinical ethics consultation and for peer review. As a consequence, Rasmussen writes that the story should contain certain core elements in order to serve as a source for review.

A common presumption in these reflections is that differences between assessments are undesirable. We disagree; indeed, we question the validity of this presupposition. In short, if clinical ethics consultation is regarded as a practice which can be understood by interpreting narratives, differences between interpretations are not in themselves problematic. A narrative approach to evaluation is based on the idea that there are no absolute standards for assessing a practice. Various stories about a practice are necessarily divergent, because they highlight various elements in that practice. The interpretations of these stories will also be different, because they departs from specific views on (the quality of) ethics consultation. This is, in fact, seen clearly in the different reviews of quality as reflected in each of the five initial peer reviews of "The Zadeh Scenario" in Part Two and the subsequent meta-reflections in Part Three. Each author, from his or her perspective, emphasizes specific elements in "The Zadeh Scenario." Stories and their interpretations can enrich our understanding of a practice exactly *because* they present various views on this practice and put the practice in a new light. Introducing a standardized approach would remove the richness of the story and its interpretations. A standardized approach is itself only one perspective, which is, like all perspectives, limited and in need of other perspectives which may complement it. Allowing for a variety of assessments may stimulate learning through a process of comparing them, and investigating where they may meet. Thus, it is the dialogue *between* interpretations that holds out the promise for actual growth in understanding what the quality of clinical ethics practice entails.

Towards a Dialogical Approach of Clinical Ethics Assessment

Several contributions to this book emphasize the need for a variety of perspectives when assessing a specific clinical ethics practice. From Frolic & Rubin, for example, we see that peer review efforts are limited and perhaps even flawed if they focus on isolated snapshots of clinical ethics practice. They write that efforts should be made to get a fuller picture through presentation of a range of narratives from the same consultant or consultation service in order to represent the spectrum of one's diverse consultations. Armstrong also argues that "*an account of the clinical engagement of a consultant is ultimately not enough to provide a holistic account of the consultant's practice, or to discern the core moral considerations that emerge among the divergent standpoints*" (Armstrong 2018: 73).

A variety of stories and interpretations can contribute to our understanding of a clinical ethics practice and its quality (Widdershoven and Molewijk 2010). This, however, requires an exchange between stories and interpretations. Putting stories and interpretations next to one another is in itself not helpful. A diversity of stories and interpretations actually calls for comparison and integration of perspectives. Various stories and interpretations can add to one another, and bring to light the limitations involved in each of them. Thus, the reviewers noticed a limitation in the Zadeh story in that the perspective of the patient is mostly absent. This implies the need for a different story, namely that of the patient. Rosell & Johnson refer to Richard Zaner in arguing for the importance of attentive interest in the patient and his/her narrative.

The value of this book is that it *shows* the relevance of stories and interpretations for assessing quality. In order to determine the quality of clinical ethics consultation, one should have in-depth insight into the actual practice of clinical ethics, which requires a multitude of stories and interpretations. Moreover, these stories and interpretations provide perspectives which are in need of exchange. A story presents a meaningful perspective on a practice, but also raises questions in the interpreter, which may require new stories in response. What is needed is a dialogue between stories and interpretations, resulting in new and richer views on the specific clinical ethics practice. Having read "The Zadeh Scenario" and the reviewers' comments, one immediately is interested in the possible answer of Finder to the reviews, and in the reviewers' reactions towards each other. Thus, stories and their interpretations call for a dialogue between the storyteller and the interpreters. As the critique of some reviewers on the absence of the patient's story shows, this dialogue should not only include the ethicist and his or her colleagues, but also other parties involved.

Responsive Evaluation as a Method for Assessing Quality of Clinical Ethics Consultation

This book contains a fine example of a narrative approach to the assessment of clinical ethics consultation quality, starting with a rich story of the ethicist about a case in consultation practice, and presenting a wide range of peer reviews and reflections. As such, it contains the basis for a dialogue between ethicists on the quality of ethics consultation, elaborating on experiences and learning from other perspectives. A next step would be to actually foster a dialogue, by organizing an exchange of stories and perspectives. This dialogue may point out the need for other stories and perspectives than those of the ethicist(s). As mentioned before, some of the reviewers suggest that the story of the patient should also be heard. Without the patient's perspective, the story about the consultation is incomplete. This is not only true for the content of the consultation (no advice can be finalized, and no valid conclusions may be definitively drawn, without taking into account the patient's wishes and concerns), but also for the assessment of the quality of the consultation. The patient's perspective is of crucial importance if it comes to determining the value of the process of ethics support. The same goes for the perspective of the family members, who were actively involved in this case.

An example of a method for assessing the quality of a practice through inclusion of perspectives and by establishing a dialogue is "responsive evaluation." Responsive evaluation actively involves stakeholders such as, in the case of moral dilemmas in clinical practice, professionals, patients and family members in evaluation to actually contribute to the improvement of concrete practices (Abma et al. 2009). It focuses on dialogical learning processes of and between stakeholders (Stake 2004; Guba and Lincoln 1989; Abma 2001; Abma and Widdershoven 2011). Responsive evaluation seeks to be inclusive and participatory: together, stakeholders determine what is good in a democratic and dialogical way (Visse et al. 2012, 2015).

Within cases like "The Zadeh Scenario," responsive evaluation can be organised in several ways. One can, for example, after the case consultation has been closed, ask the patient and the family members whether they want to reflect upon the quality of the ethics support as such. Several methods at several moments can be used. One can start with individual open interviews. Then, after having analysed the transcripts of those interviews, one can present different and similar viewpoints on what quality in clinical ethics consultation entails in a focus group interview with the stakeholders involved in the case. In the same focus group interview, or in a separate focus group, one can invite other relevant people, for instance colleague ethicists or patient and family representatives, to deliberate about the case and reflect on the quality of ethics consultation.

One way to put responsive evaluation on the quality of clinical ethics in practice is by creating a Community of Practice (CoP) (Molewijk et al. 2015; Bindels et al. 2014). Such a community is a mixed group of stakeholders (for instance, patients or their representatives, family caregivers, professionals, and ethicists) who share a common interest: the provision of good care in situations that are experienced as morally troublesome. In such a CoP, an active and explicit process of formative evaluation can take shape. By sharing analyses, experiences, and information, a CoP not only evaluates, but also improves and develops the quality of clinical ethics consultation.

Conclusion

We agree with the overall appreciation of the contributors to this book concerning the value of a narrative approach to clinical ethics consultation, both for clinical ethics consultation itself and its evaluation, as narratives present the concrete contexts in which ethics consultation takes place and the concrete individuals that are involved, and stress the subjective and action-oriented nature of clinical ethics consultation and its outcomes in clinical practice. Ethics consultation evaluation cannot be based on rules and principles that are defined beforehand, detached from concrete contexts: 'the right thing to do' is always context-bound and based on a joint reflection on lived experiences. In this sense, evaluation of ethics consultation is in line with clinical ethics practice, which also includes reflection on concrete experiences in specific contexts.

From a narrative perspective, peer review based on the ethicist's narrative account provides valuable tools to evaluate the quality of clinical ethics consultation. In addition to studying guidelines and protocols which serve as the background of a specific clinical ethics consultation service, peer review can make explicit crucial elements in consultation practice. This requires insight in what actually happens during consultation. A thick description of a consultation, such as the one provided by Finder, is of major importance for starting a dialogue on the quality of clinical ethics consultation.

This book shows that peer reviewers interpret a case narrative about consultation practice differently. This can be regarded as a sign of a lack of a common framework as a basis for evaluation, as some of the commentators do. Yet, one may also see it as an indication that evaluating a practice requires a process of interpretation in which a variety of perspectives is needed, as each perspective can add to a better understanding of what is at stake. Again, this resembles the practice of clinical ethics consultation itself, which aims at making explicit various perspectives in order to reach a better understanding of the situation at hand. Peer review is not a judgment on a practice by applying given standards, but a process of deliberation on strong and weak points of the process of consultation which is presented in the case story.

As assessment of quality is essentially a matter of interpretation and deliberation, interaction between various perspectives is crucial. The peer reviews presented in this volume call for comparison and learning to see the case better by sharing commonalities and differences. A dialogue between various perspectives will contribute to the process of evaluation, as it enables a broader view on the case under consideration. Such a dialogue should also involve the people whose practice is reviewed. All stakeholders should be enabled to bring in their perspective on the value of ethics support. Assessing the quality of clinical ethics consultation requires that the participants learn from the experiences of others, and come to joint conclusions about what is good and what can be improved.

References

Abma TA (2001) Opening thoughts. Dialogue in evaluation. Evaluation 7(2):155–163

Abma TA, Widdershoven G (2011) Evaluation as a relationally responsive practice practice. In: Denzin N, Lincoln YS (eds) Qualitative research. Sage Publications, Los Angeles, pp 669–680

Abma TA, Molewijk B, Widdershoven G (2009) Good care in ongoing dialogue. Improving the quality of care through moral deliberation and responsive evaluation. Health Care Anal 17(3):217–235

American Society for Bioethics and Humanities (2011) Core competencies for healthcare ethics consultation, 2nd edn. American Society for Bioethics and Humanities, Glenview

Armstrong K (2018) Telling about engagement is not enough: seeking the "ethics" of ethics consultation in clinical ethics case reports. In: Finder SG, Bilton MJ (eds) Peer review, peer education, and modeling in the practice of clinical ethics consultation: the Zadeh project. Springer, Cham, pp 63–73

Bindels J, Cox K, Widdershoven G, van Schayack CP, Abma TA (2014) Stimulating program implementation via a community of practice: a responsive evaluation of care programs for frail older people in the Netherlands. Eval Program Plann 46:115–121

Bruce CR (2018) Not principlism nor casuistry, not narrative ethics nor clinical pragmaticsm: a case for proceduralism. In: Finder SG, Bilton MJ Peer review, peer education, and modeling in the practice of clinical ethics consultation: the Zadeh project. Springer, Cham, pp 113–125
Dorries A, Simon A, Vollmann J, Neitzke G. 2014. The impact of an ethics training programme on the success of clinical ethics services. Clin Ethics 9: 36–44
Førde R, Pedersen R (2011) Clinical ethics committees in Norway: what do they do, and does it make a difference? Camb Q Healthc Ethics 20(3):389–395
Førde R, Pedersen R, Akre V (2008) Clinicians' evaluation of clinical ethics consultations in Norway: a qualitative study. Med Health Care Philos 11(1):17–25
Fox E, Myers S, Pearlman RA (2007) Ethics consultation in United States hospitals: a National Survey. AJOB 7(2):13–25
Guba EG, Lincoln YS (1989) Fourth generation evaluation. SAGE, Newbury Park
Janssens R, van Zadelhoff E, van Loo G, Widdershoven G, Molewijk B (2015) Evaluation and perceived results of moral case deliberation in a Dutch organization for elderly care. A quantitative and qualitative study. Nurs Ethics 22(8):870–880
La Puma J, Schiedermayer DL (1991) Ethics consultation: skills, roles, and training. Ann Intern Med 114(2):155–160
Lillemoen L, Pedersen R (2013) Ethical challenges and how to develop ethics support in primary health care. Nurs Ethics 20(1):96–108
Molewijk B, Verkerk M, Milius H, Widdershoven G (2008a) Implementing moral case deliberation in a psychiatric hospital: process and outcome. MED HEALTH CARE PHIL 11:43–56
Molewijk B, Zadelhoff E, Lendemeijer B, Widdershoven G (2008b) Implementing moral case deliberation in Dutch health care: improving moral competency of professionals and quality of care. Bioethica Forum 1(1):57–65
Molewijk B, Hartman L, Weidema F, Voskes Y, Widdershoven G (2015) Fostering the ethics of ethics consultants in health care: an ongoing participatory approach. AJOB 15(5):60–62
Pearlman RA, Foglia M, Fox E, Cohen J, Chanko BL, Berkowitz K (2016) Ethics consultation quality assessment tool: a novel method for assessing the quality of ethics case consultations based on written records. AJOB 16(3):3–14
Pedersen R, Akre V, Førde R (2009) What is happening during case deliberations in clinical ethics committees? A pilot study. J Med Ethics 35:147–152
Pedersen R, Hurst S, Schildmann J, Schuster S, Molewijk B (2010) The development of a descriptive evaluation tool for clinical ethics case consultations. Clin Ethics 5:136–141
Reiter-Theil S (2009) Dealing with the normative dimension in clinical ethics consultation. Camb Q Healthc Ethics 18:347–359
Slowther A, Bunch C, Woolnough B, Hope T (2001) Clinical ethics support services in the UK: an investigation of the current provision of ethics support to health professionals in the UK. J Med Ethics 27:i2–i8
Spike JP (2012) Training in clinical ethics consultation: the Washington Hospital Center course. J Clin Ethics 23(2):147–151
Stake RE (2004) Standards-based and responsive evaluation. SAGE, Thousand Oaks
Stolper M, Molewijk B, Widdershoven G (2015) Learning by doing. Training health care professionals to become facilitators of moral case deliberation. HEC Forum 27(1):47–59
Svantesson M, Karlsson J, Boitte P, Schildmann J, Dauwerse L, Widdershoven G, Huisman M, Pedersen R, Molewijk B (2014) Outcomes of moral case deliberation. The development of an evaluation instrument for clinical ethics support (the euro-MCD). BMC Med Ethics 15:30
Tarzian A, Wocial LD, The ASBH Clinical Ethics Consultation Affairs Committee (2015) A code of ethics for health care ethics consultants: journey to the present and implications for the field. AJOB 15(5):38–51
Visse MA, Abma TA, Widdershoven G (2012) Relational responsibilities in responsive evaluation. Eval Program Plann 35(1):97–104

Visse M, Abma T, Widdershoven G (2015) Practising political care ethics: can responsive evaluation foster democratic care? Ethics Soc Welf 9(2):164–182
Weidema F, Molewijk B, Kamsteeg F, Widdershoven G (2015) Managers' views on and experiences with moral case deliberation in nursing teams. J Nurs Manag 23(8):1067–1075
Widdershoven G, Molewijk B (2010) Philosophical foundations of clinical ethics: a hermeneutic perspective. In: Schildmann J, Gordon J, Vollmann J (eds) *Clinical ethics consultation. Theories and methods, implementation, evaluation*. Ashgate, Farnham, pp 37–51

PART FIVE
REFLECTIVE SUMMARY AND RESPONSE

Peer Review and Responsibility in/as/for/to Practice

Stuart G. Finder and Mark J. Bliton

A Beginning Thought

"I beg of you, Doctor, please don't let Dr. Moore see my mother again. My sisters and I do not want him talking with us anymore."

These opening lines of "The Zadeh Scenario" (Finder 2018: 21) foretell, in certain ways, many if not most of the core questions and themes that emerge in the ensuing layers of peer review and commentary that constitute Parts Two, Three, and Four of this volume: What is the appropriate role (and expectations and goals) of clinical ethics consultation? What are the proper goods and practices associated with actually "doing" clinical ethics consultation and hence serving as a clinical ethics consultant? More importantly – certainly for the sake of this book but also for the field of clinical ethics if it is to promote and support critical engagement among practitioners – what is the best way to capture this "doing" such that peers might be able to provide not merely critical analysis but helpful feedback and guidance? And underneath all three of these questions is yet a more basic and crucial question: what is the most appropriate frame by which we who perform clinical ethics consultation can share with and learn from each other about our performances as clinical ethics consultants – and engage in such sharing and learning as both individuals and as a field?

The opening lines of "The Zadeh Scenario" also betray; while these lines serve as the beginning of Finder's narrative, they are not, as the reader comes to learn, the beginning of Finder's involvement with Mrs. Hamadani and her family: according

S. G. Finder (✉)
Center for Healthcare Ethics, Cedars-Sinai Medical Center, Los Angeles, CA, USA
e-mail: Stuart.Finder@cshs.org

M. J. Bliton
Medical Bioethics, Kaiser Permanente Los Angeles Medical Center, Los Angeles, CA, USA
e-mail: Mark.J.Bliton@kp.org

S. G. Finder, M. J. Bliton (eds.), *Peer Review, Peer Education, and Modeling in the Practice of Clinical Ethics Consultation: The Zadeh Project*,
https://doi.org/10.1007/978-3-319-90955-4_15

to the story Finder tells, there are at least two preceding moments in time when he encountered this patient and family. First, it was in the elevator, just moments before he had his initial brief conversation with Samir Zadeh, that Finder first directly encountered members of Mrs. Hamadani's family, albeit in the typical (at least in North American cultural contexts) non-engaged style of elevator etiquette, i.e., awareness of an other's presence, but beyond a possible socially-accepted statement, such as "what floor?," no apparent (according to the narrative) acknowledgement or interaction. More remotely, as the reader also learns – and as Finder remembers upon reflection while in the midst of his initial conversation with Mr. Zadeh – he was familiar with Mrs. Hamadani and her family from prior review of "cases" which Finder and his colleagues routinely do as part of the normal functioning of the Clinical Ethics Consultation Service for which, the reader is told, Finder serves as the clinical chief and director.

But little else is provided about both of these encounters; the reader is not told, for instance, what Finder actually *did* in the elevator besides the fact that he, Samir, and Nadira (one of Mrs. Hamadani's daughters) "rode down to the bottom floor in silence" (Finder 2018: 21). Since this is the start of Finder's engagement with this family, the reader may wonder, did Finder look at them once he was in the elevator? If he did, for how long and in what ways? Did Samir and Nadira look at *him*? And were there any moments when Finder and Mrs. Hamadani's children noticed each other *looking at each other* (if in fact each did look at the other)? Or was Finder oblivious of Samir and Nadira beyond his initial noticing that they had been talking as he walked into the elevator but then ceased to talk once he was fully entered; after that, did he look at nothing in particular as the doors closed and the elevator gently glided down to the main floor? If this was the case, then the fact of what Samir and Nadira did or did not do is not something that Finder could report about, so perhaps this is the rationale for the lack of detail. The "encounter" in the elevator might have actually been less an encounter and more a mere accidental sharing of the space of an elevator moving from floor to floor.

On the other hand, given the typical experience of actually being within a confined space such as an elevator with other people, readers may wonder if Finder could have been fully oblivious; could he truly have *not* noticed such possible sensory elements as the scent of aftershave or perfume, or perhaps lingering food smells or even body odor? And what about where each stood in the elevator, how many floors it was until they reached the ground floor, and how far in front of Finder were Samir and Nadira as they, like him, walked through the lobby and out onto the plaza in front of the hospital's entrance? And did these children of Mrs. Hamadani engage in any conversation as they walked ahead of Finder, hushed murmurings that he might have slightly overheard? Or did they maintain their silence from the elevator even there in the foyer and out into the plaza?

Ordinary, everyday experiences of being in elevators or walking behind people while in public spaces often includes noticing such things; talking explicitly about them, however, is rare, possibly odd. To draw attention to them, after all, often infers evaluation – why else talk about what is otherwise left unsaid unless to suggest they are worth noting? Indeed, even here, in the above paragraph, with the mention of the *possibility* of noticing the scent of lingering food smells or body odor there is a risk of implying an evaluation since body odor in particular is rarely mentioned in ordinary, everyday interactions, including interactions that are part of clinical ethics consultation.

In "The Zadeh Scenario," there is no mention of any of these kinds of details that may have been present during Finder's encounter with Samir Zadeh. If the presence of details is typically taken to infer some sort of significance, is the *lack* of mention similarly significant, worth noting, worthy of attention? What this question elicits is what was discussed in the Introduction, namely, that determining the relevance and meaningfulness of the details of ordinary, everyday experiences requires a shift in attention, a different kind of "noticing" whereby focus is directed towards how, so to speak, thing are "lively" in the actual circumstances of their occurrence. In this light, think about what *is* presented in "The Zadeh Scenario," for example, when Samir begins that initial conversation with Finder. How striking is that encounter: Samir, whom Finder has not met, merely briefly encountered in the elevator, calls to Finder and then they are face-to-face, and Finder is called out – "I [see] on your name badge that you are the Director of Ethics and so I was thinking…" (Finder 2018, 22). This is a confrontation, not merely a conversation. With Samir's calling out to, and calling out, Finder, Finder does not know what this is about nor how it is going to go. And so, almost immediately, even as Samir finishes his sentence, Finder must pay attention in a manner that will help him assess how best to be able to respond to whatever has prompted this "calling out." The elements of such an encounter, and the assessment that unfolds, thus begin to become layered. There is, for example, the ride down the elevator and previously unnoticed pre-judgments Finder may have made but which may now emerge as significant in terms of how Finder responds. There is, in other words, a shift in attention and awareness as Finder begins to try and understand, and learn, from why Samir has stopped and confronted him. But, as the reader knows and we have acknowledged here, Finder mentions nothing about any of these potentially influential matters in his narrative as he recollects that crucial first encounter on the plaza. Is this indicative of a failing, an act of irresponsibility, a deviousness on Finder's part? Or does it reflect the challenge of describing the nuances and moral relevance of such experiences in a way that is both faithful to what transpired then and to what will come to occur later on? While "The Zadeh Scenario" offers no answers, what it does offer is that, mentioned or not, the moment of confrontation between Samir and Finder on the plaza establishes a horizon between that moment, as a moment of "here and now," *and* whatever is to come later on.

In a similar way, readers might also note that although the Scenario does report that Finder recalled his colleague, Steve Moore, telling him about Mrs. Hamadani's situation at some points in the past, beyond the sketch of that reflection – which, it also could be noted, occurs in the midst of Mr. Zadeh telling Finder his story (should the reader be worried that Finder became distracted by his own thoughts when he should have been listening attentively to Mr. Zadeh?) – the Scenario provides the reader very little information about the character and content of those conversations

Finder had with Moore. But surely *those* exchanges, as considerations about what was going on with Mrs. Hamadani and with her children that Moore encountered and reported, *they* played some role in preparing Finder (upon his recognition that this was *that family*) to not merely respond as he did but to interpret what he was doing, what they were doing, and what needed to be done going forward – all practical elements associated with judgment within clinical ethics. And yet, here too Finder offers no glimpse into these matters (nor do any of our contributors note their absence as potentially significant). And so a pertinent question might be, should Finder have told us more about this dimension of his experience?

For that matter, the readers of "The Zadeh Scenario" (be they the contributors to this book or you who now are reading this chapter, presumably after having also read the Scenario and the subsequent responses and reflections) are also not told what Finder and Moore (were there other colleagues involved as well?) discussed when Mrs. Hamadani's situation served as an example in one of the Clinical Ethics Consultation Service Reviews that is mentioned nor what had been the response to the fact, as duly referenced in "The Zadeh Scenario," that "no one [had been] willing to take the lead and more officially state, in Mrs. Hamadani's medical record or at a family conference, that continued treatment would not be appropriate, should not be pursued" (Finder 2018: 23).

All of the above is, in fact, another example of the layering and shifting of focus that is bound up with the unfurling of meaning in actual moments of engagement and interaction with others. Likewise, within the actual experience of colleagues talking about a particular clinical ethics situation, there are many details provided, some that may, at the moment of their delivery, *seem* to be relevant but turn out *not to be* given whatever subsequently happens as the consultation unfolds in the context of its actual circumstances. In fact, other details, minor at the initial time of their occurrence, come to be significant later on. And there are yet additional details, glanced or misremembered initially, that develop meaning and significance in the context of further details and events that unfold and emerge at yet still later moments. All of which is to say, clinical ethics practice, as *clinical*, is dynamic, unfolding, sometimes full of surprise, always experienced in real time, and otherwise engaging. Such is the nature of clinical ethics consultation.

"The Zadeh Scenario" does not provide a comprehensive articulation of any of these types and kinds of detail beyond the few lines about there being an encounter in the elevator and the unfurling of Finder's own recollection which interrupts Mr. Zadeh's relating his concerns to Finder at the very beginning of the narrative. As a starting point, then, for critical responses to" The Zadeh Scenario," it must be explicitly noted that there is a difference between talking about these details and layering in the actual circumstances of a specific ethics consultation and talking about them as an example of the practice of clinical ethics consultation – or even more, as an example submitted for evaluation of one's practice of ethics consultation. Understanding *why* distinguishing all of these is necessary turns out to be directly relevant to establishing a more accurate appreciation about how to evaluate Finder and "The Zadeh Scenario" – and is a significant step toward providing additional insight into how to evaluate both clinical ethics practice and the written reports or narratives that attempt to accurately describe such practice in general.

In the case of "The Zadeh Scenario," one possible reason for its not providing all of these potential details and relevant layers is something else we discussed in the Introduction to this book: the Zadeh narrative is a fragment, and as such it should not be understood nor read as a total and complete documentation of everything that Finder thought and did over the course of the 3 years since Mrs. Hamadani's situation first appeared on the Clinical Ethics Consultation Service radar (recall: the initial involvement of Moore in Mrs. Hamadani's situation began 3 years prior to the events presented in "The Zadeh Scenario"). In reading the Zadeh narrative, it would actually be quite odd for any reader to think that this narrative – or any narrative for that matter – could provide such a total and complete documentation; no piece of writing, whether fiction or memoir can contain all such details.

Indeed, as Rasmussen discussed in some depth and Bishop also amplified (Rasmussen 2018; Bishop 2018), part of the device of "The Zadeh Scenario" is that, like any ethics consultation narrative which aims to provide some description of clinical ethics practice in those ways it is actually experienced, the Scenario is necessarily limited; it is a snapshot that is now outside of time even as it strives (whether successfully or not) to capture the sense and flow of time in Finder's work. The sense of time in the narrative, moreover, like much else in "The Zadeh Scenario," is the result of construction, i.e., the writing process. In the moment when Finder enters the elevator and Samir sees him, sees Finder's name badge and Finder catches a glance but doesn't make any particular reference to it while Samir is now focused by the fact that Finder's badge says that Finder is the Director of Ethics and hence Finder may be able to intervene and do something about what Samir perceives to be the peskiness of Moore – all of that unfolds in multiple moments, even layers, of time. For example, this represents a particular time as experienced by the Hamadani children over 3 years of their mother's illness while simultaneously representing the specific focus of the palpable sense of time experienced by Finder with Samir in the face-to-face confrontation on the plaza.

Far from a mere noting of certain obvious differences between experience and *reporting on* that experience, these details discussed above highlight a crucial starting point for any serious reading of "The Zadeh Scenario" and critical reflection on what it presents: "The Zadeh Scenario," like other such narratives that attempt to capture actual moments in the practice of clinical ethics consultation, is, as an example, a piece of fiction, a story, a matter of invention. By this we mean that it contains certain details but excludes a potentially infinite set of others. And akin to how many, if not most, of the details that are presented in the Scenario are presented intentionally, so too other details have been left out with similar intention. But perhaps more importantly, many details are also left out simply due to the limits of the narrative form itself. Another limitation of "The Zadeh Scenario," in other words, is not merely that it is a fragment; it is a story, a (hopefully) coherent narrative, a piece of composition by a specific author who initially set out to achieve *something* in that activity of writing about his experience. Moreover, experience, even if fragmentary – for instance, one's beginning is also always somewhere in the middle of one's, or others', experiences writ more broadly (a point Bishop briefly addressed) – still remains different from reports about experience. Whether Finder included information in "The Zadeh Scenario" about where he was looking while in the elevator with Samir and Nadira, and whether he smelled stale food odor, and whether Samir and Nadira started to speak again once off the elevator and several yards in front of Finder as all three left the building, and any number of details about Finder's own perceptions, the environment, his thoughts, etc., in the midst of his actual experience were as they were; they occurred. And, sometimes, such occurrences turn out to be significant for the kinds of judgments one makes, for better or worse. We know that the ways others speak, appear, walk, and so forth can prompt prejudices, attractions, predispositions of various kinds that make subsequent interactions seem easier or more difficult. Similarly, in the midst of such noticing, tones of voice, word choice, fidgetiness, gestures, etc., of the other and oneself may alter how things subsequently unfold. The point here, quite simply, is that the concern for the presence or absence of details in stories is not merely about the integrity or trustworthiness of such stories; even if no story is to be told, these are the kinds of details that we routinely take into consideration when making judgments, whether it involves seemingly non-consequential judgments such as how loudly to speak (if there is some evidence of the other having difficulty hearing) to more substantive judgments (such as whether to offer one or two examples as part of an assessment of whether the other understands what one has just tried to explain). These considerations, as well as many more regarding clinical interactions, also point toward another kind of challenge associated with clinical ethics practice, namely, identifying what actually matters within those interactions with others, such that the things which *may* actually help become integrated into practice – and hence *should* be included and presented as part of peer review.

And all of the above leads to a final piece of important preliminary recognition that demands explicit notice: because stories such as "The Zadeh Scenario" (and similar efforts of clinical inquiry aimed toward representing some form of experiential truth) are constructed, created, designed, and limited, a central challenge must be addressed about how best to tell the experience of doing clinical ethics consultation in ways that accurately represent whatever might be taken as key ingredients of (and for) one's clinical ethics judgments. In other words, the methods that work best to re-present clinical activities and judgments may, even are likely to, obscure and alter key elements, including unique characteristics, actions, emotions, relationships and so on, that occurred in those moments of activity and judgment. Such are the limitations of writing.

Several of the peer reviews and commentaries acknowledged this point; we pay prolonged attention to it here because it is against this background that we must be vigilant. Indeed, the writing of this book has been inevitably framed by the kinds of inherent predispositions, prejudices, even unintentional deceptions – or if "deceptions" is too strong a term, the embedded conceits – of language. We are, therefore, keenly aware that the use of narrative devices and code words for the sake of retelling and re-presenting events via "The Zadeh Scenario" and in each of the subsequent chapters, including this one, further inevitably shapes what readers are able to "see" within what is presented. And this point, we believe, is crucial for peer review writ large, for in that effort as well, the subtleties of experience transmitted through the language used to tell and to evaluate are altered, because what emerges in that focus, its themes, and transmission, becomes as much about the practice of writing or the practice of telling (about what we do when "doing" clinical ethics) as it is about the practice of clinical work. More importantly, this book was designed to demonstrate how the core questions which undergird peer review mentioned at the beginning of this chapter – What is the appropriate role (and expectations and goals) of clinical ethics consultation? What are the proper goods and practices associated with actually "doing" clinical ethics consultation, and hence serving as a clinical ethics consultant? What is the best way to capture this "doing" for the sake of peer learning? What is the most appropriate frame by which to engage in such learning, individually and as a field? – are to be, indeed, *need* to be engaged as part of the peer review process itself.

What Exactly Does "The Zadeh Scenario" Attempt to Re-present?

It is now necessary to turn our attention toward another crucial element of the Zadeh Project, namely, the necessity for distinguishing the goals, and associated models, for doing peer review – which will directly influence how clinical practice and moral experience are to be represented. As discussed in the Introduction, "The Zadeh Scenario" was not originally written for the sake of peer review, nor was it written in order to capture every facet of Finder's interaction with Mrs. Hamadani, her three children, and the various healthcare providers involved in her care. Nor, for that matter, was it written to capture the constituent elements of Finder's clinical judgments. Rather, it was written in an extensive moment of trying to make sense of an experience, and in so doing, the effort was to create coherent moments *of* that experience of being engaged in the actual activities and interactions encountered while serving as a clinical ethics consultant. It was only after it was written, also mentioned in the Introduction, that the idea of its value for exploring issues associated with peer review emerged since, unlike narratives written for the sake of promoting a particular view of one's practice or furthering a methodological argument about how ethics consultation ought to be performed, "The Zadeh Scenario" merely aimed to try to capture something of Finder's experience, warts and all if that's what it ended up showing. In this sense, its creation was primarily concerned with capturing *something*, and that *something* being from the past; it was not, in other words, written in the hopes of pre-configuring something for the sake of the future – such as concluding that what Finder did was done well. As such, the aim of writing "The Zadeh Scenario" was neither to glorify nor condemn Finder and his practice, but to draw attention to certain experiential demands of doing the work of an ethics consultant – and then to see if there was something to be learned by turning to that experiential account again, and with others bringing their own critical perspective.

Furthermore, whether Finder was able to achieve some recognition, or not, about what was vital to the interactions depicted in "The Zadeh Scenario," what has become clear throughout the Zadeh Project are the ways that such meanings – and even a family's grief – risk becoming appropriated into other narrative forms which unavoidably make those meanings into *something else*. With specific reference, then, to what matters morally, and to what is significant to the interpretation of the values and ethical bearing of those persons actually involved, the crux of the question is whether the "*something else*" made by ethics reports, or "ethics cases," or narratives about clinical ethics encounters adequately describes "*something*" of what it was and "*something else*" of what unfolded. For Finder, the initial impetus was whether "*something else*" was going on that may have been obscured, and yet was there and *needed* to be told.

As an example, consider Finder's last encounter with Mrs. Hamadani's children and Dr. Broukhim (Finder 2018, 37–42). If one primary activity for ethics consultants is to ensure that conversational formats are available and responsive to the actual circumstances, and that the necessary processes and interactions are attempted, in order to discover those values and standpoints that are relevant and meaningful for those people directly involved, then it would seem that Finder has brought forward a key moment, a decisive moment, in the moral conversations he portrays. Indeed, what unfolds is apparently quite clear regarding Samir's understanding of his mother's situation, the medical and family choices made so far, and what looms before him and his sisters regarding their mother's medical status such that he makes one final request not to talk about all of this anymore – and to talk about *whatever* needs to be discussed only with Dr. Broukhim going forward. All of those elements, as provided by Finder, would thus *seem* to accurately represent what it is like to actually be participating in that kind of conversation. And yet, as clear as that description may be, considerable ambiguity about the actual moral understanding of each individual still remains, as does a significant degree of uncertainty about the accuracy of the different appraisals being made, right then in the moments of that encounter which Finder attempts to capture over these pages. One sort of question then, is *does* this description accurately approximate what it is like to be in that kind of situation? If not, another question is: Do we need research studies with video ethnographies and verbatims? Furthermore, and more specific to our response here, there is this primary ethical question: In the context of what has been told, why *wouldn't* Samir Zadeh's requests be fitting and morally faithful to what has been going on?

The Zadeh Project as a whole is an expansion of that last paragraph: it has been designed to be, and aims to document, a process of discovery and the variety of ways that such discovery is relevant to clinical ethics practice, and more specifically, just how such discovery is engaged in by other clinical ethics consultants, especially when reviewing practice. And yet, as discussed by many of our collaborators already, writing for the sake of evaluation – using the typical set of understandings associated with "peer review" – is a different kind of activity than writing for the sake of reporting or for the sake of discovery. If the aim of peer review is and should be evaluation – and even further, to establish (or not) an individual's satisfying some kind of professional requirement (such as may be part, for example, of a professional credentialing process) – then how an ethics consultation is represented in a written format may be quite different from what is found in "The Zadeh Scenario." The same holds for "case write-ups" that serve as part of the reporting structure within an institutional accountability framework (such as the VA's IntegratedEthics' CASES model) since the aim of that kind of endeavor differs as well from either the aim of discovery or the aim of establishing professional standing. This is a crucial point to note because it begs a critical question central to the Zadeh Project as a whole: is "The Zadeh Scenario" sufficient for probing questions regarding clinical ethics consultation peer review?

How to answer that question depends upon what, exactly, "peer review" is said to entail – a question which itself brings to light that "peer review" may be understood quite variably; examples include: evaluating an individual's performance against some established set of standards for the sake of admittance into or dismissal from a group (e.g., a professional society, a institutional staff, a practice group); determining suitability for sharing one work within a professional community (as occurs with manuscript review or presentation proposal review for professional meetings); establishing merit for the sake of having projects funded (expert panel reviews, for instance, by granting agencies); learning from an individual how he or she practices; or serving as an occasion to reflect more extensively on the practice in which peers share a commitment. While not meant to be an exhaustive or definitive list, the point is that "peer review" may refer to a variety of practices, each with potentially different aims, criteria for evaluation, format demands, etc., some of which may themselves thwart or undercut the legitimacy of the other possible aims, criteria, formats, etc. These sort of tensions are actually demonstrated by the ways that the very form and style of "The Zadeh Scenario" serve as points for critique by several authors in Parts Two, Three, and Four.

Perhaps more importantly, along with assumptions regarding the purpose of peer review and the acceptable forms for providing accounts of clinical ethics practice, there is also a wide array of substantive commitments regarding clinical ethics practice within the field of clinical ethics generally; this is wonderfully, and most explicitly, demonstrated by the chapters constituting Part Three. Demonstration of this array is also found within both "The Zadeh Scenario" and the various replies and commentaries of our collaborators; this array may be captured, and briefly explored, under the heading of two simple questions: (1) Where is Mrs. Hamadani in all this? and (2) Where are the "ethics"?

Where Is Mrs. Hamadani?

Clinical medicine has as its central focus the patient who presents him- or herself in need of help; the moral obligation to provide care thus begins with that very request for help (Pellegrino and Thomasma 1981). This understanding of the source of medicine's obligation, and thus the moral grounding of clinical practice, is ancient. Perhaps not surprisingly, a similar kind of primacy is given to the patient in discussions of the moral obligations associated with clinical ethics consultation; it is almost a kind of unspoken cardinal rule that the primary source of ethical concern within any given clinical context is patient-centric. However, just as the nature of clinical contexts are inherently dynamic due in part to the diversity of people interacting with one another from within many different roles (of which the patient is but one individual occupying but one role), the source of ethical concern in a given clinical situation may be similarly varied and diverse (Zaner 1988) – and, in fact, may primarily *not* be grounded in matters associated with the patient *per se*. Think, for instance, of situations in which different providers understand their responsibility toward a shared patient differently such that questions of intra- and interprofessional obligations are at issue. Or consider when an individual provider encounters internal moral disruption due to competing commitments – perhaps due to institutional versus professional obligations, individual versus group commitments, local versus national standards of practice, and so on – that might temporarily inhibit that individual from acting, or from acting well.

If part of the aim of clinical ethics consultation is to identify and clarify what is at stake in a given clinical situation (a point made by several of the contributors to this volume and one which we have argued in numerous publications [Bliton and Finder 1999, 2002, 2010; Finder and Bliton 2008, 2011]), then it follows that what may be demanding of attention, in that effort to discover what's going on, may not directly concern or be immediately about the patient at all. Indeed, if, for example, the locus of ethical concern is the felt sense of responsibility of a son or daughter of a patient, especially when the patient lacks the ability to interact with care providers and hence it is to the patient's children to whom care providers turn for input when crucial decisions need to be made regarding the patient's care, then so too must the ethics consultant direct attention to these individuals. Clarifying *their* sense of responsibility would thus be of central import for the ethics consultant. As such, it is not necessarily the patient *per se* who is most important even if the concern for the son's or daughter's sense of responsibility is due to something concerning the patient; in seeking to understand what matters to that son or daughter, it is him or her that is of central concern in the actual engagement of ethics consultation. Sometimes, then, it is the family, or the nurses, or the physicians, or others, to whom ethics consultants must direct their care and attention – and hence it is not merely or primarily the individual who lies in the bed that requires that focus.

Consider now what is displayed in "The Zadeh Scenario" and a recurring criticism of Finder in the subsequent commentaries: Mrs. Hamadani is peripheral, not central. More specifically, while Mrs. Hamadani's situation is the center around which events in general revolve, as Finder tells it, he seemingly did little (or perhaps even *nothing* according to some of our collaborators) to uncover *directly* Mrs. Hamadani's voice during his involvement with her family. Instead, as the critiques of Finder's practice maintain, the primary focus of his attention, and the primary voice to which he seemingly listens, is that of Mrs. Hamadani's family, and in particular, her son, Samir. Mrs. Hamadani appears to be essentially absent from the ethics consultation – a point that could have been amplified by our collaborators (we are surprised that none mentioned this so directly) by noting the very title of the narrative: it is "The *Zadeh* Scenario" – and hence *not* "The *Hamadani* Scenario."

The critical question to be asked, however, is whether Mrs. Hamadani's voice, if present *or* absent, is the *right* frame for critiquing what Finder presents in "The Zadeh Scenario"? Or, put slightly differently, why *not* focus on Samir? To be sure, the emphasis on Samir and the concerns he highlights are themselves framed by Mrs. Hamadani who, at the point that Samir confronted Finder outside of the hospital's entrance, is critically ill in the ICU, and the picture painted of Mrs. Hamadani – by her children, by her physicians, by Finder's colleague Moore – throughout the scenario is not one of an engaged, awake, alert patient. But imagine that things were different, that in the narrative Finder reported that Mrs. Hamadani *was* fully capacitated, *was* fully engaged in participating in decision-making about her care; how would that be relevant to Finder's engagement with Samir? With Nadira and Farzana? With Broukhim? With Moore? And, within a concern for practice, what is Finder actually *to do*, in the sense of actual tasks and activities as occur within institutional settings such as a hospital once Samir stops him and begins his disquisition?

Continuing with this imaginative theme, the answer, if one is to root the answer in what institutional life allows – including the institutional dimensions of clinical ethics both as locally practiced and professionally promoted (by, for instance, ASBH via the *Core Competencies* and corresponding *Education Guide* publications [ASBH 2011, 2015, respectively]) – is that it depends. The details of the situation make a difference, and with just a bit more imagination, we can fashion scenarios in which the fact of Mrs. Hamadani's capacity and her having a voice in her plan of care may have *everything* to do with the ethical dimension of how any of these involved individuals may be experiencing their felt sense of responsibility – or very *little* to do with the sense of responsibility. For instance, if Mrs. Hamadani's children are struggling to honor their mother who, they report, is being explicitly clear that they not interfere with what she has decided is best for herself – even to the point that she refuses to talk with social workers, chaplains, or others who may be interested in trying to help foster better relations between her and her children as she is now coming more rapidly to the end of her life – what would be the rationale to assert that the ethics consultant *must*, nonetheless, engage with Mrs. Hamadani even when she's explicitly requested *no* such engagement (such being duly documented in her medical record)? Or had Finder discovered, in the aftermath of Samir's initial request to keep Moore away from this situation, that Broukhim was struggling with his obligation toward Mrs. Hamadani but found his interactions with Moore to provide great moral support – not in the sense of "emotional support" (which several of our collaborators present as important but somehow diminished in import in comparison to "ethics") but in the sense of allowing for the examination and affirmation of key facets of his obligations as a care provider, i.e., Moore helped Broukhim better understand and appreciate the ethical dimensions of medical responsibility – for what possible reason would it be necessary to give voice to Mrs. Hamadani's concerns? The only plausible answer would be if Mrs. Hamadani's concerns were material for Dr. Broukhim's concerns, which *could* be the case but *need not be* the case. And if not the case, then no need to bring Mrs. Hamadani's voice into that context except insofar as to clarify what matters for Broukhim. This raises two crucial issues.

First, it seems that the argument for bringing Mrs. Hamadani's voice into this context is grounded in the presumption that clinical ethics, like medicine, must be patient-centric. If so, then this effort to hear from Mrs. Hamadani as part of the effort to lend moral support to Dr. Broukhim reflects a kind of contradiction since her input is sought for the sake of helping Brouhkim (and hence is not, *per se*, a patient-centric effort). Be that as it may, there is a second problem: to seek Mrs. Hamadani's input presumes a kind of positivity, namely that Mrs. Hamadani will not be harmed by seeking her input. But Finder does not yet know, after he has spoken with Samir and Nadira, whether Mrs. Hamadani's contribution will have a positive, negative, or neutral effect on *her*. Indeed, at the beginning, Finder lacks any context-specific criteria for even *evaluating* whether such contribution will be positive, negative, or neutral. To begin with the assertion, nonetheless, that Finder *must* give voice to Mrs. Hamadani thus seems to bring into the context a set of values or commitments that are grounded outside of this situation. Perhaps the response would be that while it is not clear at the beginning, it will become clear later on, as Finder learns more about the situation, Mrs. Hamadani, and so forth. But here too arises that possibility that seeking Mrs. Hamadani's input may turn out not to be necessary, and perhaps, even harmful.

These imaginative exercises are in no way merely academic. Rather, they reflect some elements of what is at stake in actually moving beyond the reception of a request for clinical ethics consultation into taking actual and practical steps forward into an unfolding process. A number of our collaborators make explicit appeal to the fact that clinical ethics practices are contextually bound and hence clinical ethics practitioners must be able to respond, and hence will be held accountable for such responsiveness, to what is actually going on. What "is actually going on," the ways to recognize and describe *that*, becomes the focal issue – and more importantly, the moral awareness that with any particular step forward into that unfolding future, the steps chosen are not free of value, free of commitment, free of implication for what is held as worthwhile and what, conversely, may be disregarded or deemed to be not as important or valuable or worthwhile.

With that being said, the more important point to address at this juncture of the unfolding which has occurred over the past 175 or so pages is that the assumption of patients having a privileged placement in the context of clinical ethics consultation may become problematic for evaluating the work that an ethics consultant performs as part of ethics consultation. Indeed, even if Mrs. Hamadani was fully capacitated and wanted to be fully involved in the decision-making associated with her healthcare, the apparent starting point for Finder in which he becomes more directly involved with Mrs. Hamadani's situation is Samir's stopping him and asking for his help. So, as *one* beginning point, Finder must respond to Samir and what *he* presents. What comes next will depend on what occurs there, then, at that beginning point.

In that respect, one of the factual points becomes about the "here and now" of the Scenario, that it was not Finder who chose to begin with Samir; Samir chose to approach Finder. In that moment of beginning, and going forward as well, how to understand and evaluate what Samir subsequently presents to Finder, and how to integrate that into what Finder might subsequently learn about Mrs. Hamadani and her situation, becomes part of Finder's task as ethics consultant. Finder's work as an ethics consultant thus includes being able to evaluate what is presented by Mrs. Hamadani's family. And returning for the moment to what is presented by and found within "The Zadeh Scenario," this evaluation for which Finder is responsible is to be done in the context in which Mrs. Hamadani was critically ill, in the ICU, and, based on the available medical reports which Finder reports in the Scenario, dying. It is not that being in the ICU and being critically ill and dying negate a patient from having a voice; it is that in tertiary care hospitals having ICUs, most of the patients in the ICU *have no* voice except as available through their representatives (family, formal Agents, etc.), and hence it is toward those others that ethics consultants must turn.

And this highlights a critical practice element for doing clinical ethics consultation: in actually turning attention toward these other individuals, i.e., Mrs. Hamadani's children, Finder must respond to whatever it is that they present *even if*, it turns out, what they state *is not* likely or even accurately reflective of what this patient, Mrs. Hamadani, would speak if capable. Especially at the beginning, Finder *does not know* which way it will work out and so must take as legitimate what these others present (even if also maintaining a kind of skepticism in order to assess that legitimacy). In this sense, it may be said that Finder must be *responsively* responsive when responding to what is presented to him in any given clinical ethics moment (to play off the notion, in the immediately preceding chapter, of "responsive evaluation" [Widdershoven et al. 2018: 199–200]).

As such, at least one crucial reflective point about clinical ethics consultation practice to highlight here is that once called into a situation, the ethics consultant must be prepared to address the concerns of the other individuals who accompany patients. And, such concerns are to be addressed with full intentionality and with utmost care and concern since what is presented may be an accurate representation of what the patient would speak if capable – but may not be. Furthermore, if the patient is owed some form of initial respect, so too are those others who present themselves as representing the patient even if, it subsequently turns out, what they present does *not* represent the patient. Highlighted in this way, a core ethical point about clinical ethics practice becomes evident: part of the practice is to be prepared to take into careful consideration what a family presents, and hence not only the patient (as the body in the bed and hence the focus of medical attention).

An obvious point perhaps, one we hope generates little disagreement. What is noteworthy, on the other hand, is that the details associated with the depth and extent of such careful attention, of how this is actually done and how doing so is experienced within clinical ethics practice, receives little explicit attention in the clinical ethics literature. This dearth of attention is, in fact, part of what motivated the Zadeh Project initially. More importantly for the actual practice of clinical ethics consultation, it is within the context of such moments of needing to learn from those with whom one is now interacting – especially when they are individuals with whom one has had no prior relation and hence are, for the most part, strangers – that this very practical questions gains force: "How best does one engage in the process of discovering what matters in what is going on?"

When discussing a book or a journal article or even a narrative fragment such as "The Zadeh Scenario," the form of questioning, and hence of discovering what is meant or what serves as a central point, is typically direct; one can ask simply and plainly, "what does this paragraph (or sentence or word) mean and how does it relate to whatever else the author has written?" And, this may be asked directly in part because that which is being questioned is itself partially contained between both what has been written (and hence read) so far and what is yet to be read but nonetheless still also already written – and hence already determined (in the sense that subsequent paragraphs, sentences, even words are already written, already presented, already *there*, which is what allows for *direct* examination). The same, however, cannot be said of conversations which occur in the midst of clinical ethics practice (hence another element of ambiguity associated with "The Zadeh Scenario," and with any after-the-fact "case report" that re-presents what occurred at some prior moment; *those* words, i.e., the words of the case report, and hence, for example, of "The Zadeh Scenario," are now set even as what they re-present was, at the time, not set but unfolding). Conversations, in the ways they actually occur between people, are full of uncertainties, ambiguities, and all sort of unknowns – including what may turn out to be informational mis-directions or even flat-out nonsense.

In the face of the actual uncertainty of what it is that one is encountering in the midst of having conversations as part of clinical ethics consultation, it may be suggested that such clinical interaction requires *indirection*, because being direct may not only *not* be possible (meaning is still developing, still unfolding, still being formed) but runs the serious risk of *over*-determining the meaning of what is unfolding *in* such conversations. Accordingly, clinical ethics practice has need for a kind of covert operative element, that is, something that aids in scoping out what actually matters to those individuals with whom the ethics consultant speaks. Moreover, this must occur in a manner that does not force interpretation before even initial meaning is allowed to unfurl. Hence, even the manner in which a question is asked, or a statement is acknowledged, must be done with care; the actual words chosen, and the inflection utilized when speaking those words, can make a difference in how what is said is understood by the other with whom one is speaking. The experiential dimension of "doing" clinical ethics is thus no mere secondary consideration.

Accordingly, consider how all of the above is actually performed. In "The Zadeh Scenario," some of this is demonstrated by how and where Finder meets with his various interlocutors. For instance, he goes and meets with Mrs. Hamadani's two daughters, Farzana and Nadira, in Mrs. Hamadani's ICU room. Hynds is critical of this meeting insofar it does not include all potential stakeholders, including medical authorities who may address technical questions or concerns that may arise (Hynds 2018, 90–1). On the one hand, this is a legitimate concern since the possibility is clearly present that Farzana or Nadira may ask questions about any number of aspects associated with Mrs. Hamadani's care (including insurance issues, dietary questions, and so forth; it is not merely medical expertise that is absent from the room when only Finder is there) for which Finder is unprepared, and professionally unable, to address. But the possibility of such matters arising without the needed experts being present points toward the need for the ethics consultant to know, and abide by, the limits and bounds – and hence responsibilities – of ethics consultation as practiced within the particular context. The fact of uncertainty, in other words, does not demand an avoidance of possibility. More importantly, and thus on the other hand, this concern fails to appreciate how the contexts of conversation both shapes and limits the content of such conversation. Talking with a patient's family within the confines of their domain in the hospital, i.e., the patient's room, may provide them greater comfort and hence trust as compared to bringing them to some other room for a "family meeting," the connotations of which may prevent them from speaking openly and honestly about whatever it is that they, for themselves, hold to be most significant and worthwhile.

The point here is not that ethics consultants should never meet in rooms other than patient rooms, or that ethics consultants should or should not talk with patients and their families independently of other healthcare providers. Rather, it is to raise for inspection core questions about how one might go about actually learning from patients and families about what matters most to them regarding the situations in which they find themselves as well as in some or another future into which they are headed. And in this light, Finder's going into Mrs. Hamadani's room to talk with Farzana and Nadira highlights something else: developing trust with others who are mostly strangers is as much a practical dimension of clinical ethics practice as other more typically identified skill and knowledge sets (e.g., as outlined in ASBH's *Core Competencies* document). Clinical ethics consultation thus demands a kind of deliberateness in clinical conversation, especially with patients or families, that is quite different from other kinds of engagement in which ethics consultants might participate (for instance, with ethics colleagues or administrators or members of the media). After all, whatever level of trust that may be embedded within the role of "ethics consultation" within the particular institutional context in which ethics consultation is practiced, or within the role of "ethics consultant" for those who fulfill the institutional role of ethics consultation, the *trustworthiness* of those who fulfill the role needs to be newly established for each new ethics consultation, and possibly even for each encounter within a given consultation – and this develops mostly by how and when and where those individuals occupying that role engage with others.

In summary then, rather than asking, "Where is Mrs. Hamadani?" the questions to ask are, "Whose voice should be given attention, and why?" and "How should the various voices that are present in the situation be balanced?" And equally important, "By what means should Finder have gone about discovering what matters most for each of these stakeholders given the actual dynamics of the situation as they became known?" As much as following protocols and abiding by policies, engagement in ethics consultation in the effort to answer these questions demands responding to accidental and unforeseen (and unforeseeable) factors; as Agich emphasizes in his commentary, clinical ethics consultation is a practice, and not just a body of knowledge or a set of skills (Agich 2018, 142–4). “Being responsible” in the role of “ethics consultant” is therefore not reducible to “being responsible” in the role of “ethics consultation” since the latter addresses institutional demands whereas the former focuses upon the enactment of those institutional demands within the real and dynamic contexts of actual clinical engagement with particular patients, families, clinician colleagues, etc. To “do” or “perform” or “engage in” clinical ethics consultation is thus (in part) to be continually refining and adjusting (what is being done, understood, developed, etc.) in response to what is encountered in the specific clinical situation – in which “the specific clinical situation” references both *this particular clinical situation* (as distinct from other clinical situation revolving around other patients) and *this specific moment in* this particular clinical situation. To respond as such, i.e., to refine and adjust what one is doing in response to what one is encountering (and to do so in real time), is another way of saying that ethics consultants must be responsively responsive to what they encounter.

Where Is the “Ethics”?

Responding responsively to what is actually encountered as part of clinical practice serves as an important dimension of the ethical grounds for “responsibility” in clinical ethics practice. This is no mere analytic assertion, however; the idea of responding responsively highlights the fact that even those taken for granted commitments and understandings which frame and define clinical ethics consultation itself are, potentially, available for questionings or interrogation *as part of* clinical ethics consultation. This is especially so if what emerges as significant for those individuals with whom the ethics consultant interacts raises questions regarding such commitments and understandings.

A key question, then, is what should serve as the appropriate form of analysis regarding Finder’s engagement with the sort of complexity as is found within the specific situation presented in “The Zadeh Scenario”? This question is itself complex and multi-layered – and this is independent of the important concern addressed by both Rasmussen and Bishop that peer reviewing Finder is wholly dependent upon how Finder is presented via the Scenario narrative, i.e., if Finder, the author, has done a poor job of re-presenting his actions in the “The Zadeh Scenario,” then whatever is said about “Finder” the ethics consultant within the narrative is severely limited (Rasmussen 2018; Bishop 2018). Granting that Finder’s depiction of his practice, even if fragmentary, is nonetheless accurate, the question of appropriate ethical analysis has at least three layers.

First, with Samir’s turning and stopping Finder outside the hospital doors, Finder immediately becomes a direct participant in a situation about which, at the moment of initial engagement, he knows nothing and he is, in a manner of speaking, a complete stranger, an outsider, someone who has suddenly crossed the border into a new territory, namely, the life of Mrs. Hamadani and her children. In that initial moment, the immediate question he faces is not merely how to take in and maneuver through what is now actively unfolding before him as Samir tells his tale but whether some sort of response beyond an administrative-role-based one is warranted. Finder, in other words, is at a kind of ethical juncture where he must attempt to make sense of, and evaluate, the various kinds and degrees of commitments, values, and beliefs regarding what Samir seemingly holds to be worthwhile as such are expressed by what Samir is speaking. A similar kind of evaluative effort will, of course, likely be repeated as Finder becomes more involved in the situation and thus encounters expressions of, for example, notions of felt responsibility (professional, institutional, personal) among the many individuals involved in caring for Mrs. Hamadani and interacting with her children. There will also be expressions of familial obligation bound-up in what Samir, Nadira, and Farzana tell him as well as in their understanding of love for their parents and for each other. At various junctures of encounter, Finder must assess, and possibly re-assess so as to determine what to do next.

At issue, in the moments of actual consultation activities, then, are practical considerations such as what responsibility might mean: for instance, to Samir, to Dr. Broukhim, to other providers involved in the care of Mrs. Hamadani and in the support of her children, and so on. The probing of any one of these individual's self-understanding of his or her responsibility will require some form of ethical evaluation on Finder's part as he "takes in" what each offers (whether directly or indirectly) about his or her understanding of responsibility.

In that exploration, there is then a second question about ethical analysis, namely, as Finder engages the issue of the meaning, for example, for Samir of Samir's responsibility, what kind of ethical frame should Finder utilize to assess the responsibility Finder *himself* bears in assessing Samir's responsibility? This is a potent question since how Finder understands his responsibility will shape how he engages Samir, and draws from Samir, Samir's *own* understanding of his (Samir's) own responsibility and that of Finder in turn; this is what it means, in part, for Finder to be "responsively responsive" in this situation. And whatever the frame for exploring and developing understanding of Samir's commitments, beliefs, values, and so on, Finder must also determine which to use with Broukhim, with Moore, with the others; these may be the same or these may differ – but whether same or different, if the goal of Finder's interaction with these many individuals is to discover what actually matters to them such that each sees this or that option, action, decision as better or worse, Finder's choices here are no light matter. A miscalculation in understanding runs the risk of altering the possibility of further exploring with these other individuals what actually is at stake for them, information that is necessary (even if not sufficient) for Finder's ability to help in the situation.

And with all that said, there is at least, then, a third layer of ethical assessment, namely, that which is to be utilized by Finder's peer reviewers – especially if the presentation Finder provides (via "The Zadeh Scenario," for instance) is divergent from typical norms of "ethics consultation" (for instance, that a patient's voice is paramount). For Finder's peer reviewers, to not take up this third layer of assessment (i.e., their own frame for evaluating Finder's practice) as part of their engagement with the narrative and then their evaluation of Finder runs the serious risk of misunderstanding what Finder may be trying to present in his narrative – akin to Finder risking misunderstanding, for instance, what Samir presents in Samir's presentation (including his initial confrontation with Finder outside the hospital doors or in the meeting in which he, his sisters, Finder, and Broukhim had which is recounted near the narrative's end). And so a fourth layer emerges as well: what kind of ethical analysis is at stake not merely for Finder's peer reviewers but for the process of peer review itself?

Given the above, it is curious to note that through-out Parts Two, Three, and Four, the idea that "The Zadeh Scenario" lacks any evidence of ethical analysis, that Finder offers no account of "ethics" in his narrative, is repeated. This claim, however, may be said to be more a reflection of presumptions by our collaborators about what counts as "ethical analysis" – and hence the subject of the third layer described above – than what Finder presents or does. Indeed, it may be argued that the entirety of the Scenario is an exemplification – as opposed to a didactic description – of at least the first two layers of ethical concern described above. And taken together with the critiques lobbied against Finder, this entire book is explicitly, but as an indirection, raising the question of the fourth layer, as a form of critical engagement. So while we agree that "ethics" as typically discussed in didactic texts is nowhere to be found in "The Zadeh Scenario," it is, we believe, everywhere evident in the story told, in the responses to that story, and in the subsequent responses to the responses. Once again, therefore, we return to the notion of unfolding and the idea that meaning and responsibility in the actual practice of clinical ethics consultation, as experienced by those who serve in the role of clinical ethics consultants, is to be, at least in part, discovered through the process of engagement with others.

Drawing to a Close: Learning for the Sake of Improving Practice

In the opening paragraph of this chapter we noted that underneath the core questions and themes that emerged in Parts Two, Three, and Four is a more fundamental and crucial question facing those who engage in clinical ethics consultation practice, namely, what is the most appropriate frame by which to share with and learn from each other regarding the actual performances as clinical ethics consultants – and then, by extension, how best to engage in such sharing and learning not merely individually (as might occur among immediate colleagues within a given clinical ethics consultation service) but also as a field? On the one hand, the very structure of this book explicitly reveals much about what we, the collective authors of this book, take to be necessary in that effort: one must be willing and able to attempt to capture an account of one's clinical ethics practice experience. One must be further willing to put such representation of one's performance before others for the sake of discovering what cannot be discovered on one's own, i.e., being committed to collaboration as key for developing self-understanding. One must also be willing to collaborate with others from a breadth of backgrounds and perspectives regarding the practice of clinical ethics – and thereby be willing to accept that diversity in clinical ethics practice should be sought, not eliminated. In addition, that experience, accounting for experience, critiquing experience and critiquing accounts of experience are neither interchangeable nor reducible to each other nor mutually exclusive. And finally, we take as necessary that the ethical dimensions of clinical practice, clinical experience, clinical reporting, and the review of each are grounded in such experience, practice, and accounting – and hence not originating from what may be outside or beyond the limits of the clinical.

With all that being said, on the other hand, the aim of the Zadeh Project, beginning back in at least 2009 when the initial idea of putting together that first panel in which the Zadeh narrative was presented for colleagues to then critique, has also always been to raise questions for the sake of challenging whatever presumptions and pre-conceptions we, and our collaborators, may bring into the Project; this includes presumptions about not merely whatever may be more directly revealed (or hidden) in the Zadeh narrative itself but also as regards clinical ethics practice more generally as well as clinical ethics method, clinical ethics training, and efforts to professionalize the clinical ethics field. The structure and content of this book, therefore, has been designed to equally challenge and promote – and in the process, offer an account of *that* practice. Rather than write a book that offers didactic direction regarding the process and role of peer review and peer learning as pertains to clinical ethics practice, we have sought to display it and to leave for you, the reader, the ensuing questions not merely to ponder, but to incorporate in whatever account of peer review you (and we) might subsequently build, locally for our own individual clinical ethics consultation services and as a field.

As such, there is another set of fundamentally ethical considerations with which we are committed – but which we are as yet unwilling to challenge – and that is the centrality of affiliation and trust as central grounds upon which clinical ethics consultation practice must rest. Through-out this book, the themes of affiliation and trust have been present, whether it is within the relational dynamic of Finder and Moore, Finder and Broukhim, Finder and Samir Zadeh, Samir and Farzana and Nadira, Broukhim and Mrs. Hamadani's children, Finder and all five authors in Part Two, those authors and the authors of Parts Three and Four, or all of us who have collaborated in this book and you the reader. At each level, there is something shared, something trusted, something ingredient to clinical ethics practice.

Whatever else may be found within "The Zadeh Scenario," one thing that stands out is an expression of multiples forms of obligation that texture and shape clinical encounters. There are obligations of healthcare providers: to patients, to the family members who accompany their patients, to clinical colleagues, to their institution, to their profession. There are obligations of family members: to their loved one the patient, to each other as family and those who care about the patient (even if not directly providing care to that patient), to those who provide care to their loved one the patient, to their community that extends beyond family and patient in which their lives have been and will continue to be lived. And there are obligations of professions, of institutions, and of communities in which patient, family, and healthcare providers may interact beyond the healthcare context that also are brought forth into clinical contexts, sometimes intentionally, sometime explicitly, oftentimes only by presumption. In many instances, those presumptions are difficult to find, difficult to understand, difficult to manage because, for the most part, most who are brought together by a particular patient's situation – patient and family, on the one hand, and healthcare providers on the other – are strangers in each others' worlds, which itself raises questions about responsibility each may bear in the face of that shear, and mundane, fact. Whatever else clinical ethics consultation may, or must, address, this fact cannot be overlooked if the aim of clinical ethics, even nominally, is to address what may serve as the source of ethical tensions, conflicts, and disruptions revolving around a patient's care.

And this brings us full circle to the issue of fragment, because any form of giving an account is fragmentary – and "fragmentary" as defined by any number of political, professional, institutional, cultural, etc., criteria in light of which the issue of understanding and evaluation occurs. And this holds true not merely within the context of discrete clinical interactions but also for any form of peer-to-peer engagement, most especially when what is at issue is institutional/professional understanding and evaluation. So, in the end, the question raised by several of our collaborators regarding "The Zadeh Scenario," namely, does it present an "ethics" consultation at all, may be the penultimate question to consider. In ways it is and in ways it is not. It is surely an example of clinical ethics support, and there was awareness and alertness to many of the aforementioned factors of affiliation and trust in the activity of actually staying in conversation in and with the situation, which represents a kind of inquiry that is ingredient and essential to clinical ethics consultation. To be sure, again as various collaborators have highlighted, within the scenario there was not mention of any formal analysis; the primary focus was to support the family and physicians in what was unfolding in the care of this patient, Mrs. Hamadani, as she lay dying. At the deepest layer, then, is the question of what ethics "consultation" is to mean when the kind of engagement revolves around the moral dimensions of patients care, dimensions in which ethical analysis may be possible (from a distance) but not necessarily asked for or fitting in the moments of engagement.

At stake is therefore the very question of ethics and of consultation in the meaning and commitments associated with clinical ethics consultation. Peer review thus becomes an occasion not merely of vetting who can pass as an ethics consultant worthy of that moniker but for critical engagement within the field regarding the question of ethics and of consultation. Peer review is, in other words, yet another means for peer learning about what we in the field hold to be of fundamental value. But it is not enough merely to state those values; they must be enacted in the very "doing" that is clinical ethics practice. And similarly, they are to be found in what we present to, and seek from, our peers.

Peer review, in the context of peer education, rests upon a commitment to model – and demands engagement with – what is most worthwhile for the practice and the field of clinical ethics. This book has attempted to lay out some of the commitments that we, the collective authors of this book, share – and question – including the need to provide accounts, seek critique and guidance from peers, and to consider the implications of such critiques. Such efforts, of course, are in some sense, never completed as the very engagement will, inevitably, lead to more questions. But that is part of the goal, part of what is sought, for in the emergence of new questions arises the opportunity to learn, to reform, to move (hopefully) forward into something improved; whether it is an improvement, of course, remains to be seen.

This chapter began with the acknowledgement that foretold in that first encounter Finder had with Samir Zadeh are many if not most of the core questions and themes that subsequently emerged in the ensuing layers of review and commentary that constitute Parts Two, Three, and Four. Now at the end of the chapter, and at the conclusion of the Zadeh Project (as it is captured by the pages of this book), we here return to those core questions, only now as transformed through a process of recognition, identification, appraisal, clarification, and evaluation:

How might one be responsible *in* clinical ethics practice?
How might one be responsible *as* a clinical ethics consultant?
How might one be responsible *for* the practice of clinical ethics consultation?
How might one be responsible *to* the field of clinical ethics?

We leave these questions with you, the reader, in the hopes that you will take them up and come to discover something of significance for not merely what you do if you "do" clinical ethics consultation, but how, and why, to engage in peer learning and peer review – for yourself, for your immediately colleagues, for the broader set of colleagues with whom you regularly interact while fulfilling whatever the local institutional expectations of "ethics consultation" may be, for administrators who need to know why what you do is worth supporting, and for the field as it continues to develop into whatever it is that "ethics consultation" will come to mean going forward. We have attempted to model a way of doing so, one that entails providing imaginative variations of experience, reflection, response, and exploration. The task is now yours.

References

Agich GJ (2018) Narrative and method in ethics consultation. In: Finder SG, Bliton MJ (eds) Peer review, peer education, and modeling in the practice of clinical ethics consultation: the Zadeh project. Springer, Cham, pp 139–150

American Society for Bioethics and Humanities (2015) Improving competencies in clinical ethics consultation: an education guide, 2nd edn. American Society for Bioethics and Humanities, Glenview

Bishop J (2018) Doing well or doing good in ethics consultation. In: Finder SG, Bliton MJ (eds) Peer review, peer education, and modeling in the practice of clinical ethics consultation: the Zadeh project. Springer, Cham, pp 179–192

Bliton MJ, Finder SG (2002) Traversing boundaries: clinical ethics, moral experience, and the withdrawal of life supports. Theor Med Bioeth 23(3):233–258
Bliton MJ, Finder SG (1999) Strange, but not stranger: the peculiar visage of philosophy in clinical ethics consultation. Hum Stud 22(1):68–97
Bliton MJ, Finder SG. 2010. A Brief Reflection on the Experience of Responsibility in Ethics Consultation. Formosan J Med Humanit 11(1&2): 93–102
Finder SG (2018) The Zadeh scenario. In: Finder SG, Bilton MJ (eds) Peer review, peer education, and modeling in the practice of clinical ethics consultation: the Zadeh project. Springer, Cham, pp 21–42
Finder SG, Bliton MJ (2008) Responsibility in actual practice: consent and participation in clinical ethics consultation. In: Hester M (ed) Ethics by committee: a textbook on consultation, organization, and education. Rowman & Littlefield, Lantham, pp 79–106
Finder SG, Bliton MJ (2011) Responsibility after the apparent end: 'following-up' in clinical ethics consultation. Bioethics 25(7):413–424
Hynds J (2018) Ethics consultation, professional praxis, and what it means to be a "consultant". In: Finder SG, Bliton MJ (eds) Peer review, peer education, and modeling in the practice of clinical ethics consultation: the Zadeh project. Springer, Cham, pp 85–97
Pellegrino ED, Thomasma DC (1981) A philosophical basis of medical practice: toward a philosophy and ethic of the healing professions. Oxford University Press, New York
Rasmussen L (2018) Standardizing the case narrative. In: Finder SG, Bliton MJ (eds) Peer review, peer education, and modeling in the practice of clinical ethics consultation: the Zadeh project. Springer, Cham, pp 151–160
Widdershoven G, Molewijk B, Metselaar S (2018) Peer review and beyond: towards a dialogical approach of quality in ethics support. In: Finder SG, Bliton MJ (eds) Peer review, peer education, and modeling in the practice of clinical ethics consultation: the Zadeh project. Springer, Cham, pp 193–203
Zaner RM (1988) Ethics and the clinical encounter. Prentice-Hall, Inc., Englewood Cliffs (Reprinted in 2002 by Academic Renewal Press)

MIX
Papier aus verantwortungsvollen Quellen
Paper from responsible sources
FSC® C105338

If you have any concerns about our products,
you can contact us on
ProductSafety@springernature.com

In case Publisher is established outside the EU,
the EU authorized representative is:
Springer Nature Customer Service Center GmbH
Europaplatz 3, 69115 Heidelberg, Germany

Printed by Libri Plureos GmbH
in Hamburg, Germany